Global Reflections on COVID-19 and Urban Inequalities series

Series Editors:

Brian Doucet, University of Waterloo
Rianne van Melik, Radboud University
Pierre Filion, University of Waterloo

This timely four-volume Shorts series explores the challenges and opportunities facing cities in the wake of the COVID-19 pandemic. Offering crucial insights for reforming cities to be more resilient to future crises, this is an invaluable resource for scholars and policy makers alike.

Titles in the series:

Volume 1: Community and Society

Volume 2: Housing and Home

Volume 3: Public Space and Mobility

Volume 4: Policy and Planning

Find out more at:
https://bristoluniversitypress.co.uk/global-reflections-on-covid-19-and-urban-inequalities

EDITED BY
RIANNE VAN MELIK, PIERRE FILION,
AND BRIAN DOUCET

VOLUME 3: PUBLIC SPACE AND MOBILITY

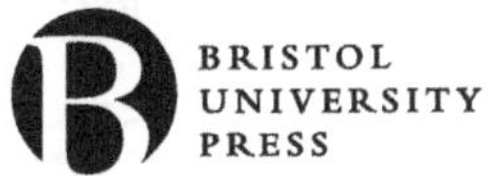

First published in Great Britain in 2021 by

Bristol University Press
University of Bristol
1–9 Old Park Hill
Bristol
BS2 8BB
UK
t: +44 (0)117 954 5940
e: bup-info@bristol.ac.uk

Details of international sales and distribution partners are available at
bristoluniversitypress.co.uk

British Library Cataloguing in Publication Data
A catalogue record for this book is available from the British Library

ISBN 978-1-5292-1900-5 hardcover
ISBN 978-1-5292-1901-2 ePub
ISBN 978-1-5292-1902-9 ePdf

Cover design: blu inc, Bristol
Front cover image: E4C/istockphoto.com
Bristol University Press uses environmentally responsible print partners.
Printed in Great Britain by CPI Group (UK) Ltd, Croydon, CR0 4YY

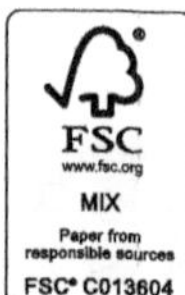

Contents

CONTENTS

List of Figures

Notes on Contributors

Aamstrong Anjumuthu is an architect and independent researcher in India.

Emma Arnold is a Postdoctoral Research Fellow at the Department of Sociology and Human Geography at the University of Oslo, Norway.

Luce Beeckmans is an Assistant Professor in Architecture and Urbanism related to Migration and Diversity at Ghent University and a Senior Postdoctoral Research Fellow at the Flanders Research Foundation, Belgium.

Rubén Casas is an Assistant Professor at the School of Interdisciplinary Arts and Sciences at the University of Washington Tacoma, US.

Alice Corble is an Academic Services Supervisor at University of Sussex Library, UK.

Mattias De Backer is a Postdoctoral Researcher at the KU Leuven Institute of Criminology and the University of Liège Centre for Ethnic and Migration Studies, Belgium.

Harya S. Dillon is the Secretary General of the Indonesian Transportation Society, Indonesia.

Phuong Quoc Dinh is the Course Director (Interior Architecture) and a Lecturer at the School of Design, Swinburne University of Technology, Melbourne, Australia.

Julian Dobson is a Senior Research Fellow at the Centre for Regional Economic and Social Research, Sheffield Hallam University, UK.

Brian Doucet is an Associate Professor and Canada Research Chair in the School of Planning at the University of Waterloo, Canada.

Arlinde Dul is a Master of Science (Faculty of Spatial Sciences) and Master of Arts (Faculty of Arts), University of Groningen, the Netherlands.

Lígia Ferro is a Researcher at the Institute of Sociology and Assistant Professor at the Faculty of Arts and Humanities, University of Porto, Portugal.

Pierre Filion is a Professor at the School of Planning of the University of Waterloo, Canada.

Alexandra Flynn is an Assistant Professor at the Allard School of Law, University of British Columbia, Canada.

Neluka Leanage is a consultant specializing in active transportation and a PhD Candidate at the School of Planning, University of Waterloo, Waterloo, Canada.

Ute Lehrer is a Professor at the Faculty of Environmental and Urban Change, York University, Canada.

João Teixeira Lopes is a Researcher at the Institute of Sociology and Professor at the Faculty of Arts and Humanities, University of Porto, Portugal.

Anastasia Loukaitou-Sideris is a Distinguished Professor of Urban Planning and Associate Dean of the Luskin School of Public Affairs at University of California – Los Angeles (UCLA), US.

Setha Low is a Distinguished Professor of Environmental Psychology, Anthropology, Geography, and Women's Studies and Director of the Public Space Research Group at the Graduate Center of the City University of New York (CUNY), US.

Loren March is a PhD Candidate at the Department of Geography and Planning, University of Toronto, Canada.

Peter Massini is a green infrastructure practitioner and policy maker in the UK.

Louise Meijering is a Professor in Health Geography at the University of Groningen, the Netherlands.

Lucas Melgaço is a Professor of Urban Criminology at the Vrije Universiteit Brussel, Brussels, Belgium.

Phuong Thu Nguyen is a PhD Candidate at the School of Economics, Finance and Marketing at Royal Melbourne Institute of Technology, Australia.

Stijn Oosterlynck is a Full Professor in Urban Sociology at the University of Antwerp, Belgium, and Chair of both the Centre for Research on Environmental and Social Change and the Antwerp Urban Studies Institute, Belgium.

Tess Osborne is a Researcher and Lecturer in the Faculty of Spatial Sciences at the University of Groningen, the Netherlands.

Lakshmi Priya Rajendran is a Senior Research Fellow in Future Cities, Anglia Ruskin University, UK.

Júlia Rodrigues is a Research Fellow in the CRiCity project at the Institute of Sociology, University of Porto, Portugal.

Deden Rukmana is Professor and Chair of the Department of Community and Regional Planning at Alabama A&M University, Alabama, US.

Nicholas A. Scott is an Associate Professor of Sociology at Simon Fraser University, Vancouver, Canada.

Eunice Castro Seixas is a Researcher at the Research Centre in Economic and Organizational Sociology (SOCIUS), and the Principal Investigator of the CRiCity project at SOCIUS, Lisbon School of Economics and Management, Universidade de Lisboa, Portugal.

Ha Minh Hai Thai is an architect and urban designer in Vietnam and Australia and Lecturer at the School of Architecture and Urban Design at Royal Melbourne Institute of Technology, Australia.

Amelia Thorpe is an Associate Professor in the Faculty of Law and Justice at the University of New South Wales, Sydney, Australia.

Rianne van Melik is an Assistant Professor at the Institute for Management Research, Radboud University Nijmegen, the Netherlands.

Meredith Whitten is an Economic and Social Research Council Postdoctoral Fellow at the London School of Economics and Political Science, UK.

Conor Wilson is a PhD candidate and Associate Lecturer at the School of Business and Creative Industries, University of the West of Scotland, UK.

Anaid Yerena is an Associate Professor at the School of Urban Studies at the University of Washington Tacoma, US.

Acknowledgments

This volume is one of four in the Global Reflections on COVID-19 and Urban Inequalities series, edited by Brian Doucet, Rianne van Melik, and Pierre Filion. The editors of this series would like to thank Bristol University Press, in particular Emily Watt and Freya Trand, for their help and guidance while working with us to publish these books quickly. Thanks to Helen Flitton and Anna Paterson from Newgen Publishing UK for their detailed and timely work on copy-editing and production. We would like to thank the anonymous reviewers of our series proposal, as well as the individual manuscripts for their helpful and constructive feedback. We would especially like to thank Brayden Wilson, an MA student in Planning at the University of Waterloo, for his coordination of the administration of this project, including his frequent and thorough correspondence with over 70 contributors that helped to keep this project on schedule. Brayden's work was supported thanks to funding from Canada Research Chairs program, under award number 950-231821.

Territorial Land Acknowledgment – Brian Doucet and Pierre Filion work at the University of Waterloo and reside in the City of Kitchener, which are situated on the Haldimand Tract, land that was promised to the Haudenosaunee of the Six Nations of the Grand River, and is within the traditional territory of the Neutral, Anishinaabeg, and Haudenosaunee peoples.

Preface to All Four Volumes of Global Reflections on COVID-19 and Urban Inequalities

You are currently reading one of the four volumes of Global Reflections on COVID-19 and Urban Inequalities, which jointly explore schisms the pandemic has both revealed and widened, and measures taken to mitigate or eradicate these societal gaps. The aim of this series of edited volumes is to bring together a collection of critical urban voices across various disciplines, geographies, and perspectives in order to examine the urban challenges of COVID-19 and its impact on new and existing inequities in cities around the world.

There are two sides to the pandemic. As a highly contagious disease, given enough time and a lack of effective mitigation to restrain its spread, COVID-19 will eventually infect a large majority of the population, regardless of income or geography. This is why many public health measures are directed at entire national (or indeed global) populations. But we have also quickly learned that COVID-19 is selective in its effects – for instance, based on age and comorbidity – and that the pandemic and responses to it exacerbate fault lines traversing cities, societies, and, indeed, the world order.

There is a clear urban dimension to these inequities. Some parts of the city and some populations who reside in cities are more likely to contract and spread the virus. COVID-19 is thus an amplifier of pre-existing social divisions. Access to medical treatment and possibilities to physically isolate from potential infection are unevenly distributed. So too are the consequences of policy responses, such as lockdowns, the economic impacts of the pandemic, and the individual and political reactions it prompts. The pandemic has therefore increased divisions such as between young and old, rich and poor, left and right, and countless other societal dichotomies. As a result, experiences of urban life during the pandemic vary greatly. Where these impacts of the pandemic intersect with pre-existing racism, ageism, sexism, ableism, and spatial divisions within the city, the consequences have been particularly severe. As we write this preface, vaccines are starting to be produced, distributed, and administered. This poses new questions: will we emerge from the pandemic thanks to these vaccines? How equitable will the distribution of vaccines be within countries and at the global scale?

This context suggests myriad potential urban futures. The planning, policy, and political choices made in the short term will impact the medium- and long-term trajectories of cities and the lives of their residents. Moving forward, the challenge is how to ensure that planning and policy responses to the pandemic do not further exacerbate pre-existing inequalities and injustices that were amplified because of COVID-19. Therefore, there is a need for engaged, critical urban scholarship in order to ensure that issues of social justice and equity are front and center, not only in academic debates, but in rapidly evolving planning, policy, and public discussions that will shape these urban futures. Our four volumes suggest pathways that can help make this possible.

Rather than speculate, however, this book, and its three companions in our series, unites well-informed, reflective, and empirically grounded research from around the world to contextualize the new and amplified inequities brought about by COVID-19. The divisions that are apparent during the pandemic are not treated in isolation; they are firmly situated as part of long-term trends and broader narratives about cities, places, communities and spaces.

Critical urban research during the pandemic

The first accounts of the novel coronavirus that would become known as COVID-19 emerged late in 2019 in Wuhan, China. Over the first months of 2020, the virus spread around the world. On March 11, 2020, the World Health Organization declared a global pandemic. Schools and businesses closed, office workers were told to work from home, and public spaces were shut. International travel came to a virtual standstill. Varying degrees of lockdown restricted the movements of people outside of their homes. In public, keeping distance from others and wearing facemasks became the norm. While the exact timing of these measures varied by country, by the summer of 2020, the majority of the world's population had experienced most of them. While the lockdowns did 'flatten the contagion curve', as restrictions of movement and activities were lifted, after a period of relative stability, infection rates took off again in the fall of 2020 and into 2021, reaching levels much higher than those experienced during the first wave.

As academics, we transitioned our own work during this time by setting up home offices, switching our teaching to online platforms and adapting our research methodologies. The specifics of our own research shifted as it became impossible to study contemporary cities without assessing the impact of COVID-19. The more we examined our own research, however, it became apparent that the key questions and approaches driving our work remained central to interpreting this new reality. The inequities we were already examining in housing, transportation, public space, metropolitan regions, and planning systems took on new dimensions because of the pandemic. But most of the inequalities that are so central and visible during the pandemic were themselves not new; they were building, in different ways, on the pre-existing inequalities of cities before COVID-19. It soon became clear that COVID-19 was exacerbating and amplifying existing socio-economic and spatial inequities, even more than it was creating entirely new ones.

The pace of change during the pandemic poses a particular dilemma for researchers, who usually benefit from sufficient time to reflect and analyze. On the one hand, jumping too quickly to conclusions leads one to speculate rather than reflect, 'opinionate' rather than research. Academics are not journalists, and it is not our task to provide real-time accounts and assessment of change.

On the other hand, as critical urban scholars, we must contribute to the discussions about the myriad ways COVID-19 is reshaping urban spaces and the lives of their inhabitants. Critical voices are more important now than ever, especially since cities face such uncertain futures and the responses to the pandemic will shape cities and urban life for years to come. COVID-19 has created urban challenges unprecedented in our lifetime. The pandemic has torn back the curtain on uneven social, spatial, and racial processes of urbanization that were previously downplayed in mainstream planning and policy debates. They have rendered visible some of what was previously invisible.

This context also gives rise to new possibilities and ideas that were once at the fringes of urban debates, such as closing streets to cars, which have been put into practice in cities around the world. But again, critical scholarship and research is necessary in order to study to what extent these planning and policy responses to the pandemic play a role in impacting (and potentially augmenting) the inequalities and injustices that are central to cities in the 21st century.

In short, it is simply not possible for urban researchers to 'sit this one out' while the dust settles. While academics may prefer to conduct research after the fact, this may be years into the future and after many important decisions have long been made. The challenge is therefore to strike a delicate balance between a slower, contemplative, and reflective approach to scholarship, while still striving to influence broader, rapidly evolving debates. We believe that our approach to this edited series strikes the right tone between these two important approaches.

The development of this edited series

Specifically, this four-part collection emerged from a meeting between our editorial team – Brian Doucet, Rianne van Melik, and Pierre Filion – and Bristol University Press in April 2020, wherein we were asked to assemble a rapid response book dealing with cities and the COVID-19 pandemic. As an editorial team, our approach has been to balance the need to make active contributions to rapidly shifting debates, while also reflecting on the impact the pandemic was having on urban inequities. We decided that short chapters, highly accessible to a diverse audience of scholars, students, professionals, planners, and an informed public, would be most suitable. The short nature of these chapters means that they fall somewhere between a typical media piece and a full-length peer-reviewed article.

A broad call for chapters was launched in mid-June 2020. Throughout various listservs and on social media, we invited researchers to reflect on how COVID-19 has impacted new and existing inequalities in cities throughout the world. We welcomed chapters that dealt with any urban topic and featured perspectives and voices not always central to mainstream scholarly, planning, or policy debates, including some co-written by non-academic authors.

The response to our invitation was overwhelming. We received many more abstracts than containable in a single volume. After a rigorous evaluation of the abstracts, we invited selected researchers to write full chapters. Keeping the best of these chapters we found ourselves with a sufficient number of chapters for four volumes. The volumes were organized around the four main themes dominating the submitted chapters.

Given the edited nature of the book, the global scale of its chapters and the wide scope of its object of study, there are inevitable gaps in the coverage of events relating to the

ONE

Introduction

Rianne van Melik, Pierre Filion, and Brian Doucet

The virus which causes COVID-19 is an invisible threat that has hugely impacted cities and their inhabitants in numerous ways, as also outlined in other volumes in this series. Volume 1 focused on how pre-existing inequalities within society have augmented and exacerbated when they have intersected with the pandemic; Volume 2 expanded on this theme with a specific focus on housing. Yet, though the virus itself might be imperceptible, its impact is sometimes very visible, perhaps most so in urban public spaces and spaces of mobility, which are the central themes of this third volume. Since March 2020, cities all over the world have restricted the access to, and use of, public spaces, in order to prevent the further spread of COVID-19 (Honey-Rosés et al, 2020). In countries with very strict lockdowns, this resulted in empty streets and marketplaces, and spatial and temporal restrictions limiting the frequency, duration, and reach of outdoor visits.

Although such restrictions generally applied to everyone, they have nevertheless rendered socio-economic inequalities along spatial lines sharper and clearer. Indeed, as Moore (2020) puts it, 'the division between the private and public space is being played out in this bizarre inability to acknowledge that

",

many do not have private outside space: that they rely on a communal "outdoors" that is now to be avoided and policed'. As such, the COVID-19 crisis added a third process producing the often proclaimed 'end' or 'death' of public space, as emphasized by Van Eck et al (2020: 375): 'In addition to the privatisation and commercialisation of public spaces, health-related regulations by local governments impact the nature of public spaces as important meeting places.' Consequently, 2020 has been proclaimed as the 'year without public space'.[1]

Yet, while at the start of the pandemic public space was considered a threat to urban health that needed to be avoided and restricted, gradually this representation shifted towards the acknowledgment that public spaces are critical infrastructures for the operation of cities (for example for access to health services and food and resource distribution) as well as the physical, mental, and emotional well-being of their inhabitants (UN Habitat, 2020). Cities as diverse as Milan, Paris, Bogotá, and Vancouver (see Chapter Sixteen, this volume) transformed previously car-oriented streets into spaces specifically assigned to cyclists and pedestrians, so that people could commute, exercise and relax while keeping their physical distance (see also Volume 4, Chapter Four). Social distancing circles appeared in parks over the world (Figure 1.1) to manage crowds having a picnic or sunbathing. Indoor sports activities moved to parks, sidewalks or even parking lots, when it became clear that the risk of contagion was smaller outdoors. Restaurants extended their business on sidewalks. However, such 'pandemic pop-up infrastructures' were certainly not distributed evenly over cities, favoring some places and peoples over others, as Flynn and Thorpe (Chapter Three, this volume) demonstrate.

Once the first wave of lockdowns was gradually curtailed in the late spring and summer of 2020, public spaces worldwide appeared to be more popular than ever. In many cities people returned to parks, (shopping) streets, and beaches in large numbers, sometimes resulting in overcrowded situations in which it proved practically impossible to keep enough distance.

Figure 1.1: San Francisco under quarantine

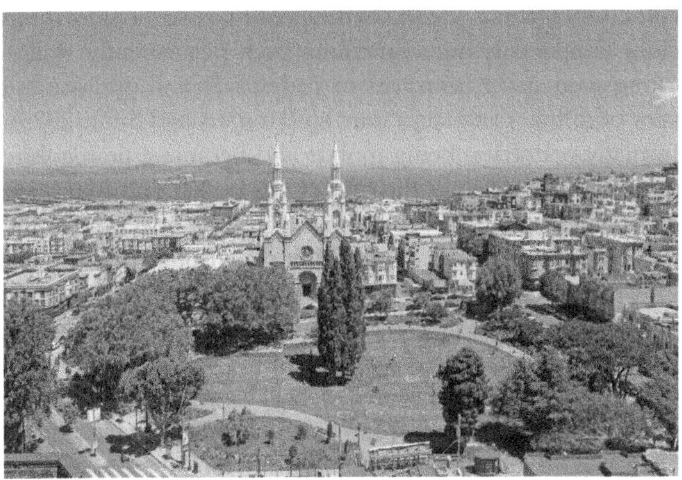

Source: Christopher Michel, Creative Commons

For example, in the Netherlands, the 'Social Distancing Dashboard'[2] has produced city maps showing how physical constraints such as the width of footpaths make it practically impossible to respect a minimum of 1.5-meter distance in historic city centers such as Amsterdam. Major events in both public and private space in the summer and fall of 2020 were cancelled in most countries, which ironically prohibited the fourth edition of the 'We Love Public Space Festival'.[3] Nevertheless, many (spontaneous) gatherings still occurred in public space and brought large crowds together, for example concerning the Black Lives Matter protests.

Following Manual Castells, we can look at public space as *space of places* (where we meet, socialize, exercise), but also as *space of flows,* or passage (to get from A to B). The pandemic resulted in major changes in our mobility behavior. Vehicle traffic reduced worldwide on our streets during lockdowns and, as we discussed in the introduction to Volume 1, public critique this development, as it often goes without any form of public participation and favors some places and peoples over others: 'While pandemic pop-ups imply a limited temporality to respond to the crisis, the infrastructure prioritized in these "pilots" sends a striking message as to which issues, and whose voices, matter.'

Beeckmans and Oosterlynck (Chapter Four) agree that in the public debate on urban life in the (post-)COVID-19 city a 'White' middle-class perspective is often dominant. Although some changes like car-free streets and more walkable cities undoubtedly will result in healthier and liveable cities, they also reconfirm a gentrification agenda that in all likelihood will not improve live for all urban dwellers equally. They hence provide lessons to also take 'non-privileged perspectives' into account.

In a similar vein, De Backer and Melgaço (Chapter Five) illustrate how the pandemic has had much harsher effects on vulnerable groups such as migrant youth, refugees, asylum-seekers, undocumented migrants, and homeless, for whom the use of public space is a necessity because they simply cannot go elsewhere as shelters were closed or overpopulated. Increased policing to enforce COVID-19 measures has perhaps made public spaces safer in terms of health regulation, but has simultaneously made them more desolate, dangerous places for homeless or undocumented women.

Dobson (Chapter Six) also talks about 'the persistence of privilege, even in spaces that are apparently equitable' when he describes how parks in Sheffield offered outdoor relief to some, like youth loitering at the General Cemetery, but certainly not to everyone, exemplified by the absence of people with disabilities or mobility difficulties.

Public spaces are the daily glue by which we come into contact with diverse and different people, which is now under threat as we behave as gated community residents shunning the 'dangerous other' (Low and Smart, 2020). Wilson (Chapter Seven) describes how the pandemic results in a re-evaluation of what is considered good or bad behavior in public space in the UK during the lockdown. He illustrates how the term 'covidiots' quickly infiltrated the lexicon of public discourse amid condemnation of those seen to be using parks, beaches, and other public spaces in spite of the UK 'stay home' imperative. However, this form of 'non-compliance' should rather be seen as a failure by design than a failure of the individual deliberately violating the rules, as access to outdoor space is not equally shared in the neoliberal city. Wilson hence urges the need to 'consider the situated, and context-specific nature of lockdown transgressions'.

Yerena and Casas (Chapter Eight) therefore conclude that public open space is fundamental to the production of just cities which promote health and wellness among residents, especially during public health crises. Like the other chapters in Part I, Yerena and Casas also fundamentally question what public space is, in their case by focusing on the link between parks and public health. This connection between public space and human well-being is further explored in Part II of this volume.

Part II Public Space and Human Well-Being

Public space undoubtedly provides benefits to the city. Streets, squares, and parks are important structuring elements of the urban landscape. They are places for unexpected encounters and public discourse as well as for relaxation and passage (Madanipour et al, 2014). The vicinity of green public space is said to benefit both real estate prices and people's health: people recover more quickly, have lower blood pressure and less muscle tension in green environments (De Vries et al, 2003). Lastly, parks and other green spaces can increase the sustainability of cities by improving air quality, decreasing traffic noise and reducing urban heat. Though these values of public spaces were long acknowledged prior to COVID-19, green public spaces, in particular, are now being rediscovered (Hospers and Smit, 2020) as critical infrastructures for the physical, mental, and emotional well-being of people.

Whitten and Massini (Chapter Nine), for example, describe how COVID-19 has led to the acceleration of existing policy plans to make London greener and more liveable. Like other contributors, they also show how the pandemic has brought existing inequalities into sharper focus, as increased park use was mostly driven by young and wealthy residents, while other less privileged population groups lacked access to a private garden or high-quality park. Yet, creating more conventional parks is difficult in a dense city like London; hence, the city now focuses on building an equitable network of green civic spaces.

Low and Loukaitou-Sideris (Chapter Ten) also stress how the built environment, and in particular its public spaces, can influence people's health, especially of older adults. The consequences of physical distancing and social isolation are adding to their anxiety and loneliness. Low and Loukaitou-Sideris therefore introduce four principles of the allocation of public space that privilege the old and most vulnerable citizens in parks and on public transit.

Osborne, Dul and Meijering (Chapter Eleven) also focus on older adults and their experiences of urban space in the COVID-19 lockdown. They found that the elderly in the UK and the Netherlands, in response to perceived risks of crowds, often chose to be in, and interact with, spaces at a short distance from their homes. Though this reduced mobility and hyperlocal everyday life might seem restricting at first, it could also facilitate 'aging-in-place' in the long term, as the elderly become more familiar with their immediate surroundings.

Corble and van Melik (Chapter Twelve) discuss the public library in the UK and the Netherlands as an important social infrastructure that not only offers access to books and information but also to social networks and care, especially for certain vulnerable groups such as people suffering from loneliness, illness, or disability. They sketch a 'crisis-upon-crisis situation', where the closure of libraries during lockdowns and only partial reopening thereafter worsened an already precarious situation for public libraries after more than a decade of austerity and budget cuts. As such, the vital role libraries can fulfill as a social contract is at risk.

Rodrigues, Ferro, Teixeira Lopes and Castro Seixas (Chapter Thirteen) focus on the contribution of public space to the well-being of children. They describe how children's independent mobility and use of public space were already declining prior to the pandemic, with urban childhood increasingly revolving around indoor settings including the home and school. Their observations of playgrounds in Porto before and after the lockdown reveal that children now engage more in solitary play, isolated from peers. As such, they might be playing outdoors again, but they are not playing together.

Rajendran and Anjumuthu (Chapter Fourteen) also discuss the implicit yet critical role public spaces play in the quality of everyday life in Indian cities. Focusing on streets as quintessential public spaces serving multiple, intertwined purposes, they show how social distancing was extremely challenging. Indian streets play a vital role in place appropriation and engagement, offering opportunities for developing and negotiating people's identity and feelings of belonging.

Thai, Dinh, and Nguyen (Chapter Fifteen) raise another contribution of public space to human well-being, that is a financial one. As also outlined by UN Habitat (2020), public space is important for the livelihoods of the urban poor, for example street vendors in Hanoi, Vietnam. The chapter illustrates the initiatives these traders employed amid the COVID-19 restrictions to generate income and provide affordable food and critical services to low-income families, like switching to forms of mobile trading after outdoor markets were closed.

Part III Mobility and Public Space

The pandemic resulted in major changes in our mobility behavior. Scott (Chapter Sixteen) uses the metaphor of a 'double-edged sword' of people's changed mobility behavior as

Hospers, G-J. and. Smit, M.J.G. (2020) 'Zo verandert corona onze steden: De gevolgen van de pandemie voor de openbare ruimte'. *Actuele Onderwerpen*, 84, July 2020.

Low, S. and Smart, A. (2020) 'Thoughts about public space during COVID-19 pandemic'. *City & Society*, 32(1): np.

Madanipour, A., Knierbein, S. and Degros, A. (2014) *Public Space and the Challenges of Urban Transformation in Europe*. New York: Routledge.

Mitchell, D. (2017) 'People's Park again: on the end and ends of public space'. *Environment and Planning A: Economy and Space*, 49(3): 503–18.

Moore, S. (2020) 'This crisis has changed our experience of home – and exposed the deep pain of poor housing'. *The Guardian*, April 6, 2020.

Sorkin, M. (1992) *Variations on a Theme Park: The New American City and the End of Public Space*. New York: Noonday Press.

UN Habitat (2020) *UN-Habitat Guidance on COVID-19 and Public Space*. https://unhabitat.org/sites/default/files/2020/06/un-habitat_guidance_on_covid-19_and_public_space.pdf

Van Eck, E., van Melik, R. and Schapendonk, J. (2020) 'Marketplaces as public spaces in times of the COVID-19 coronavirus outbreak: first reflections'. *Tijdschrift voor Economische en Sociale Geografie*, 111(3): 373–86.

van Melik, R. and Spierings, B. (2020) 'Researching public space: from place-based to process-oriented approaches and methods', in V. Mehta and D. Palazzo (eds) *Companion to Public Space*. New York: Routledge, pp 6–26.

PART I

What Constitutes Public Space?

TWO

Public Space and COVID-19:
New Social Practices,
Intensified Inequalities

Loren March and Ute Lehrer

Introduction

The pandemic itself, its rippling repercussions, and the measures to control its spread, have dramatically altered our ways of life and how we behave in public space. The production of public space, which, in our understanding is the result of social practices of people in combination, and response to, regulations and cultural norms, is undergoing major transformation. By now, we can see that these new regulations for how to physically distance in space lay bare, in fact exacerbate, already existing urban inequalities and social differences. In addition, we have experienced local waves of global social uprisings and witnessed local manifestations of resistance to safety measures themselves, all of which have important implications for what a 'new normal' might be. Planning for what constitutes public space, where its location should be, and how it ought to be managed and maintained have become a central part in what many now call a 'new normal'.

which cause nuisance or injury to other people, damage to property, or that interfere with the enjoyment of space by others. New emergency measures modified existing rules to require compliance with physical distancing. In some cases, as with physical distancing, ordinary spatial practices were forbidden (such as being within a two-meter distance of another person from outside your household), whereas in others, such as a moratorium on the eviction of encampments in public parks, existing rules were temporarily loosened. These early safety measures saw physical public spaces become heavily regulated, with many new guidelines being visibly marked out. Moving through the world and navigating social encounters became spatial practices affectively steeped in anxiety and fear of contagion.

More recently, though, as the city enters into new, optimistic phases of 'recovery' and 'reopening' (while the threat of the virus still lingers) we see experimentation on the planning and policy side of public space that seeks to enact long-term changes. In terms of urban design, we observe the City adopting new planning guidelines that enable physical distancing in public parks and on sidewalks. Alongside an encouragement of outdoor recreation and leisure activities, we notice the fast-tracking of bike lanes and of licensing for outdoor patio spaces for bars and restaurants (see Chapter Three, this volume). As the province of Ontario has gradually been 'reopening', we have seen planners and policy makers scramble to adapt 'business as usual' to the 'new normal'. A large part of this has involved appropriating swaths of public space, such as sidewalks and streets, and to occupy them with patios, restaurants, terraces, and sidewalk sales without much public consultation (the assumption being that these new consumption spaces are inherently for the 'public good'). What started first as a more makeshift approach turned into the so-called 'CaféTO program' with rules and regulations. These temporary spaces currently occupy a kind of gray area, much like privately owned public spaces (POPS) or pop-up DIY urbanist playscapes, forcing us to reconsider private-public binaries. While the fate of such spaces is unclear, their presence in the landscape sets an important precedent in terms of prioritizing private spaces of consumption in public space.

While much of this exploratory and innovative planning has trained its attention on transforming privileged and already amenity-rich spaces in the downtown, the pandemic has disproportionately impacted the 'forgotten densities' (Pitter, 2020) of the city's social and spatial peripheries. We note a glaring absence of meaningful targeted and urgent planning of 'emergency' public space and active transit corridors that might help areas like Toronto's disinvested inner suburbs, which have seen the highest levels of exposure to COVID-19 in the city, and which could use bicycle lane options similar to the downtown neighborhoods, particularly in light of reductions in public transit. Further, the urging of urbanites into city parks for recreational activities and simultaneous lifting of tent eviction moratoriums in public spaces encourage the displacement of growing encampments of unhoused Torontonians that have proliferated throughout the city during the pandemic. Activists and advocates have also sounded alarms around the over-policing and surveillance of marginalized and racialized people in public spaces during the pandemic (Canadian Civil Liberties Association (CCLA), 2020). These place-specific examples not only illustrate the ways that safety measures, planning, and enforcement must be viewed through a lens of difference but also urge us to examine public space as a socially produced space.

Emergent practices, publics, and the social production of the 'new normal'

Understanding public space as something that is socially produced encourages us to ask different questions about it. Who is urban space for? As new spatial practices emerge, and new ways to enforce particular norms, whose practices are to be adopted or encouraged? Who has power to surveil and enforce norms? Planners must remain aware that, while a friendly and sanitized discourse of park provision, recreation, and bike lanes may sometimes prevail, as our new social space is shaped, multiple publics, power imbalances, disciplinary carceral logics, and demands for justice continue to be at play. We see vast differences between how some public space is maintained and curated for a privileged public, while other public space must be claimed by counter-publics, such as protesters decrying the surveillance, policing and killing of Black people in our cities. When we discuss public space in the context of the (post)-COVID-19 'new normal', we consider the ways that diverse spatial practices and emergent, contested norms constitute that 'new normal', and thus produce public space as a multifaceted, complex, and shifty social space wherein 'distance' has many meanings.

Within what we might see as a period of radical openness, wherein norms and practices have shifted both dramatically and radically, we can see different publics pushing for changed ways of being in the world. These struggles are visible in the streets. As the pandemic's unevenly distributed impacts laid bare systemic inequities, the early months of summer saw Toronto's streets, parks, and other public spaces appropriated also for demonstrations, sit-ins, and protests. As the pandemic has continued, we have seen ongoing protests and uprisings in the streets, many large in scale, in response to systemic racism, police brutality, unsafe working conditions (most recently in relation to education), the housing crisis, homelessness, and the looming threat of mass eviction. These protests seek systemic changes and are using public space to be seen and heard. They are rooted in longstanding inequities and in problems Toronto faced long before the pandemic. Emergent publics have made claims to physical urban space in order to demand power to shape social space and everyday life in the city. At the same time, ongoing anti-government demonstrations have been attended by 'anti-maskers' and 'anti-lockdown' protesters who have largely argued that public health precautions encroach on their individual freedoms.

What is the 'new normal' taking shape through the emergent practices of various publics? The pandemic has, in upsetting the seeming stability of life as usual, assembled new publics, reconfigured existing ones, and given rise to innovative spatial tactics, triggering the opening of a space of widened possibility. In the grayness and uncertainty of this period we see openness, and highlight emergent spaces of radical potential. Where public space is concerned, we notice the opportunity to generate a 'new normal' that is not entirely centered around the maintenance of distance from one another, but instead upon recognizing mutual vulnerabilities and coming together to work collectively around questions of social transformation, justice, and redistribution. Amid a proliferation of calls for more and safer public spaces, we spot a pressing need for new visions of what public space might be. Questions of public space, for us, are thus not limited to important aspects like equitable provision of and access to physical urban spaces, but extend to the social production of urban space more broadly.

Out of the wreckage wrought by the pandemic, we see emergent practices of commoning and care that, while they have been necessitated by years of disinvestment in social infrastructure and the rollback of state supports, draw upon traditions and ethics of mutual aid from past radical movements, demonstrate the power of collectives, and provide sites of coalescence for new publics while generating new socio–spatial practices and ways of being with transformative potential. From very early on in the pandemic we have seen many individuals participate collectively in the production of 'caring infrastructures' (Morrow and Parker, 2020), delivering food and groceries to urban dwellers who were unable to enter public spaces, volunteering in and provisioning supplies for homeless encampments, or opening accessible community fridges on public city streets for those in need. The necessity for sustained collective gathering in the face of numerous injustices

March, L. and Lehrer, U. (2019) 'Verticality, public space and the role of resident participation in revitalizing suburban high-rise buildings'. *Canadian Journal of Urban Research*, 28(1): 65–85.

Morrow, O. and Parker, B. (2020) 'Care, commoning and collectivity: from grand domestic revolution to urban transformation'. *Urban Geography*, DOI: 10.1080/02723638.2020.1785258

Murray, N.A. (2020) 'The dangers of privatizing public space'. *StreetsBlog NYC*, July 5, https://nyc.streetsblog.org/2020/07/05/op-ed-the-dangers-of-privatizing-public-space/

Pitter, J. (2020) 'Urban density: confronting the distance between desire and disparity. *Azure*, April 17, www.azuremagazine.com/article/urban-density-confronting-the-distance-between-desire-and-disparity/

Schindler, S. (2020) 'Expanded outdoor dining must make space for public in public spaces'. *Portland Press Herald*, May 19, www.pressherald.com/2020/05/19/maine-voices-as-cities-move-to-expand-outdoor-dining/

THREE

Pandemic Pop-Ups and the Performance of Legality

Alexandra Flynn and Amelia Thorpe

Introduction

Cities around the world have rushed to respond to the COVID-19 pandemic by regulating public space to promote social distancing and stimulate economic recovery. The resulting decisions are what we term 'pandemic pop-ups' – hasty, real-time, and temporary changes to the use and regulation of public space. Focusing on Toronto, Canada, and Sydney, Australia, we argue that pandemic pop-ups extend beyond immediate infrastructure needs to how cities govern generally. Pop-ups may replace cars with bikes or extend restaurants into streets, and for this they have been celebrated: for saving jobs, and for making streets safer and more enjoyable. Pandemic pop-ups are not universally positive, however. They also remove tent encampments, make racialized residents more vulnerable to sanctions, and rush through controversial infrastructure projects.

As we consider pandemic and post-pandemic cities, the governance of pop-ups demands critical scrutiny. The laws that regulate urban space are always open to multiple interpretations (Cover, 1983). The force of law depends on its social context, on the ability of legal actors to give effect to their preferred interpretations and the lack (or inability) of others to challenge those interpretations. Through pop-ups, cities enact a particular form of legality – by which we mean not just legal texts, but the range of rules, practices, and understandings through which those texts take effect in the world – that weakens democratic oversight and participatory processes. With an emphasis on speed over process, pop-ups have invariably been deployed without oversight or engagement, and rarely involving the voices of racialized or vulnerable people.

We recognize the value that pop-ups can bring to cities – socially, economically, and environmentally – as well as the urgent challenges that make pandemic pop-ups critical. In this chapter, however, we focus on more troubling aspects that have often been overlooked. To do this we challenge two features that are conventionally associated with pop-ups: their irregularity and their scope. First, most accounts describe pop-up planning as exceptional, a deviation from usual practices of decision-making. Yet in the time of COVID-19, pop-ups are the 'new normal'. Second, we argue that pop-up infrastructure is broader than previously acknowledged, extending beyond bike lanes and patios to homeless encampments and policy proposals. Since pandemic pop-ups re-shape public space and the regulations through which it is governed, decisions must be made within a framework of inclusive and participatory decision-making.

What we think when we think about pop-ups

Pop-up planning is typically associated with small-scale, time-limited interventions in public space (Lydon and Garcia, 2015). Pop-ups can be used to 'minimize costs, refine designs, and gain political, public, and financial support in the creation of people-oriented public spaces' (Peterson, 2012: 2). Celebrated examples emphasize sociability and sustainability: the plastic chairs that preceded the permanent pedestrianization of Times

Square in New York; the shipping container bars and disco washing machines that led post-earthquake rebuilding in Christchurch; the weekly closures of streets to cars in Bogotá that inspired Sunday Streets around the world.

Cities are increasingly using pop-ups as soft strategies to test and build support for change while engaging citizens in ways that are more participatory than standard forms of consultation. They provide nimble processes that can be useful in overcoming resistance, enabling the replacement of infrastructures that 'have proven to be dysfunctional' (Peterson, 2012: 1). But the promise of long-term change cannot be assumed, as pop-ups often remain small and experimental. Participation is also uneven, and may minimize – or even eliminate – public engagement. Among the celebratory rhetoric, pop-ups have thus attracted critiques: for the unevenness and precarity of interventions, and for their implication in processes of displacement, gentrification, and state disinvestment (Thorpe et al, 2017).

The legalities of pandemic pop-ups

The COVID-19 pandemic has seen an explosion of pop-up infrastructure. After an initial focus on minimizing infection (allowing health and other key workers to avoid public transport by cycling to work; preventing crowds in outdoor recreation areas), the emphasis has increasingly been on enabling economic activity (allowing businesses to work with social distancing by extending their activities into public spaces).

The rapid reallocation of traffic space for walking, cycling, and dining has generated much applause, with commentators celebrating these shifts as the start of long-term change toward more liveable, sustainable, and inclusive cities (Martin et al, 2020; see also Chapter Sixteen, this volume). Yet, in the early haste to respond, some governments overlooked public participation altogether. For example, in the United Kingdom, some municipalities created cycling lanes and wider sidewalks using only technology-based data and without community

Beyond bike lanes

Pandemic pop-ups extend beyond cycling and dining spaces. Toronto is not just overlooking areas of disadvantage, but worsening them, by dismantling homeless encampments, restricting public spaces, and introducing fines that shape new social distancing regulations, disproportionately affecting vulnerable and marginalized communities (Luscombe and McClelland, 2020). By contrast, thousands of mainly White, affluent people who breached social distancing rules in a trendy Toronto park received only warnings (Van Wagner and Potamianos, 2020).

In the early days of the pandemic, Toronto grouped access to public space, cycling, and sidewalk use with the need for 'permanent supportive and affordable housing opportunities' (City Council, 2020a). Toronto initially allocated emergency shelter spaces in community centers and schools, as well as provided rooms in hotels and interim housing for the most vulnerable (City Council, 2020c). But, unlike patios and cycling, approval for these pop-up spaces expired at the end of June 2020 without a plan or funding to address where people would go later. In May and June, the City cleared tent encampments from public spaces even without sufficient housing and shelter space, and high rates of COVID-19 in the housing provided, resulting in legal action by the Canadian Civil Liberties Association (Van Wagner and Potamianos, 2020).

In Sydney, there were numerous housing-related interventions, but not the increase in funding for the construction of social housing desperately needed after decades of disinvestment. The emphasis was instead on emergency measures: temporary accommodation (hotel rooms for 30 days) and outreach services for rough sleepers and, more controversially, cash grants of $25,000 to encourage renovations by middle-class owner-occupiers 'to help the residential construction market to bounce back' (Australian Government, 2020).

The planning process itself was another focus of pop-up activity. The state government explained: 'We've brought forward immediate reforms to the planning system to support productivity, investment and jobs during COVID-19. Our plan will cut red tape and fast-track assessment processes to boost the construction pipeline' (DPIE, 2020). Introduced as part of an Emergency Measures Bill in March, these developer-friendly changes followed years of unsuccessful (and extremely unpopular) efforts to downgrade assessment and consultation processes in the planning system. The 2020 changes included increases to lapsing periods, existing use rights and appeal rights for applicants, significantly reducing the ability of local councils to regulate development. The Minister also gained new powers to authorize development 'without the need for any approval under the Act or consent from any person' (DPIE, 2020). Within two months, fast-tracked approvals were granted to 48 projects worth over $13 billion. Only some changes to the planning process were time-limited. Legislative requirements to make development proposals publicly available in council offices and to place notifications in local newspapers, for example, have been permanently removed (despite an official acknowledgment of the equity implications of online-only notification and exhibition (DPIE, 2020)).

Pandemic legality: towards a new conceptualization of pop-ups

Cover (1983: 4) writes, 'We constantly create and maintain a world of right and wrong, of lawful and unlawful, of valid and void.' Pop-ups give physical form to particular understandings about rightfulness, lawfulness, and validity, and in doing so they work to produce and preclude particular kinds of legality and precarity. Law provides the basis for multiple narratives through which 'right' and 'wrong' are produced and known;

the success of particular narratives depends upon practices of compliance, rejection, and adaptation.

Just as pop-ups can be understood as deviations from normal processes, pandemic pop-ups can be conceptualized as including new ways of enacting laws, such as delegating power for development proposals and fast-tracking long-term plans. In our view this is a central feature – and concern – of pandemic pop-ups. With pandemic pop-ups extending far beyond the usual bike lanes and patios to less convivial decisions on housing, tent encampments, and participatory planning, this is a concern in urgent need of attention. The similarities between Toronto and Sydney are significant, indicative of the proliferation of pandemic pop-ups in western liberal democracies, and reflective of the increasing globalization of actors, processes, and pressures on cities.

Cover reminds us that what is right or wrong is not merely an issue of formal law – legislation and judicial decisions – but is co-created by communities, in which a wide range of legal actors (elected officials, bureaucrats, citizens, and others) may resist and recast state-sanctioned laws. Toronto's decision to group together the public realm and housing, and then to abandon housing and destroy encampments, illustrates the continuous mishmash of legalities and the state responsibilities they entail.

Pandemic pop-ups have significant implications for democratic urban governance, especially inclusive and participatory decision-making. As we move from short-term health to longer-term economic objectives, the importance of these issues is increasingly apparent. In limiting engagement, prioritizing particular pop-ups (patios to promote business activity, major project approvals to spur development) over others (housing for those in need), and treating vulnerable communities differently, pandemic pop-ups undermine the decades of hard work to make local decision-making more democratic, equitable, and inclusive. While pandemic pop-ups imply a limited temporality to respond to the crisis, the infrastructure prioritized in these 'pilots' sends a striking message as to which issues, and whose voices, matter. Pandemic pop-ups map a set of laws that respond to only a subset of pandemic needs, and simultaneously produce gaps in democracy.

References

Australian Government (2020) *Fact Sheet: Homebuilder*, June 18. https://treasury.gov.au/sites/default/files/2020-06/Fact_sheet_HomeBuilder_0.pdf

City Council (2020a) *City of Toronto Response and the Ongoing Management of Emergency City Business during the COVID-19 Pandemic*, April 30. City of Toronto, CC20.2.

City Council (2020b) *Cycling Network Plan Installations: Bloor West Bikeway Extension & ActiveTO Projects*, May 28. City of Toronto, CC21.20.

City Council (2020c) *Ending Homelessness During a Pandemic: Calling for Immediate Action from the Provincial and Federal Governments*, June 29–30. City of Toronto, MM2217.

Committee for Sydney (CFS) and DPIE (2020) *Public Space Ideas Competition Kit*, July.

Cover, R.M. (1983) 'The Supreme Court, 1982 term-foreword: nomos and narrative'. *Harvard Law Review*, 97: 4–68.

Department of Planning, Industry and Environment (DPIE) NSW (2020) *COVID-19 Response and Recovery*, June 12. www.planning.nsw.gov.au/Policy-and-Legislation/COVID19-response

Eskyte, I. et al (2020) 'Out on the streets – crisis, opportunity and disabled people in the era of COVID-19: Reflections from the UK'. *ALTER, European Journal of Disability Research*.

Faruqi, O. (2020) 'Compliance fines under the microscope'. *The Saturday Paper*, April 18.

Lovelace, R., Talbot, J., Morgan, M. and Lucas-Smith, M. (2020) 'Methods to prioritise pop-up active transport infrastructure'. *Findings*, https://doi.org/10.32866/001c.13421

Luscombe, A. and McClelland, A. (2020) *Policing the Pandemic Mapping Project*, www.policingthepandemic.ca

debate on urban life in the (post-)COVID-19 city a 'white' middle-class perspective is often dominant. As a result, the diversity of spatial needs and the varying degrees of spatial poverty are not sufficiently taken into account. We then move on to document the impact of COVID-19, and the measures to counter it, on precarious groups living in the city. Finally, we suggest a few socio-spatial lessons which could be drawn from the lockdown for a more equal post-COVID-19 city.

COVID-19 and the city through the prism of 'urban flight'

The impact of the lockdown on urban life and the use of urban space was instantaneous. A remarkable feature of several early newspaper articles on COVID-19 and in Flemish cities and Brussels is its framing in terms of 'urban flight'. In the articles, COVID-19 is framed as a potential new driver of urban flight and thus a threat to the renewed popularity of cities with (a part of) the middle class. One article reports on the 'anguish of urban life under COVID measures […] with a small balcony or small garden, the playground fenced off with police tape and the parks where you are chased away from sitting on a bench' (Renson, 2020) and links this to a future acceleration of urban flight of 'young families' (read: 'White', middle class families). The report of a 15 to 21 percent rise of house sales in the months after the (first) lockdown – with a marked preference for houses with a garden – by the Flemish television news underscores this view (Braekman and Hofman, 2020). Much of the public debate on the post-COVID-19 city that has since followed, often unwittingly adopted this middle-class frame by focusing specifically on how to protect and recover the spatial assets that fueled gentrification in the past years, namely qualitative urban space, traffic free zones, bike lanes, and proximity to services.

This middle-class perspective on the post-COVID-19 city is also reflected in professional debates about the (post-)COVID-19 city between Flemish urban planners.

As human mobility was extremely restricted, 'unnecessary' movements by car discouraged, and the use of public transport limited to those with no other options, many started walking and cycling in their own neighborhood (Van Acker, 2020). While discovering 'hidden' parks or enjoying running on abandoned urban boulevards, urban planners (re-)invented concepts such as: the '15-minute city' in which all essential services and work is within a 15-minute walking distance from home (VRP, 2020), 'car free streets' or 'play streets' where children can safely play for instance in the absence of nearby parks (Boie, 2020; see also Chapter Eighteen, this volume).

Although all of these ideas for the (post-)COVID-19 city are undeniably valuable, they do not address the urgent socio-spatial needs of the most vulnerable urban social groups during the pandemic. Or phrased differently, while these 'best practices' in post-COVID-19 urban planning will without doubt contribute to a healthier and liveable city, they often reconfirm a gentrification agenda that will in all likelihood not improve life for all urban dwellers, especially not for vulnerable groups. The latter group does not have the 'luxury' of choice in the urban housing market – for example the 'exit' option of urban flight, but paradoxically its needs and concerns are less visible in public and professional debates on the post-COVID-19 city.

Reinforced urban inequalities under COVID-19

At first sight, the measures taken to stop the spread of COVID-19 are strict, but apply universally to each and every citizen. However, the socio-spatial living conditions of people under lockdown differed greatly. For many vulnerable people in the city, it was extremely difficult to comply with the COVID-19 measures to 'stay home', for instance due to the small size of the house, its location in a neighborhood with little open and green space, the lack of (access to) a garden, the high number of people in the house, the precarious (mental) health condition of the people, or the limited access to information and communication technologies (see also Volume 2: Housing and Home). The Belgian lockdown during the first COVID-19 peak (which included the prohibition to sit in public space) was a flat measure that applied to everyone equally, thus neglecting that certain groups are highly dependent on public space for their (mental) well-being, such as youngsters, especially those living in small apartments with no outdoor space. For this latter group with a high spatial poverty, already before the pandemic urban squares functioned as an extension of their living room (Delepeleire, 2020).

Consequently, it is important to acknowledge the heterogeneity of people to which COVID-19 measures are applied specifically from the perspective of their vulnerabilities. On top of this, COVID-19 seems to reinforce existing health inequalities, with low-income groups running a higher risk of being contaminated with COVID-19 (Bruzz, 2020; De Smet, 2020). In Brussels for example, low-income groups have a 167 percent excess mortality compared to 90 percent for higher-income groups, with lower housing conditions and pre-existing health inequalities being offered as important explanatory factors. In addition to the gradations of spatial poverty mentioned in the previous paragraph, which are most extreme for homelessness and undocumented people, there also exist a diversity of spatial needs. Some of the urban dwellers are simply dependent on the city as a survival- and social mobility 'machine', for instance for all those (neglected) that gain an income from informal labor, or the many (registered and sometimes unregistered) taxi-drivers, night shops, car washes, who do not have the choice to stay home because they otherwise have no income.

Apart from the measures that applied universally to every citizen, but impacted more heavily on vulnerable groups due to their uneven housing conditions, some (proposed) measures privileged high-income groups over others. An example is the highly charged debate on the 'secondary residents', that is, citizens with a second, holiday home at the Belgian coast or other tourist areas in the country. Some of them argued that the lockdown, which forbids non-essential travel to other parts of the country, violated their property rights (Nieuwsblad, 2020). They received a lot of public attention and support from mayors of coastal municipalities, some of whom proposed to introduce a 'beach pass' which allowed access to the beach on the basis of property rights (possessing a house in one of the coastal cities) or payment of taxes (thus also including those with a second home at the Belgian coast). The proposed 'beach pass' thus privatized a public space, that is, the beach. Similarly, the possibility given to bars and restaurants to extend their businesses into the public space (including the beach) in order to allow for more sitting places on safe physical distance regulated access to public space on the basis of consumption.

Towards a more equal (post-)COVID-19 city?

In this section, we will draw some urban (planning) 'lessons' from the earlier observations regarding the socio-spatial needs of those hit hardest by the COVID-19 measures (see also Volume 4: Policy and Planning). These socio-spatial 'lessons' work towards a more equal (post-)COVID-19 city and thus break with a prevailing discourse which departs from the perspective of more privileged urban dwellers and the fear that they may use the 'exit' option of urban flight if urban governments do not center their needs and concerns in their policies. We will start with the most private urban space, namely housing, to move to public space, which especially for badly housed groups functions as an extension of the home. We will end with a discussion of a semi-public space, that is, health care facilities, of which COVID-19 showed the need to re-center it, socially as well as spatially, in the operation of disadvantaged neighborhoods to effectively counter health inequalities.

Research has shown that there is no correlation between population density and the spread of COVID-19, but that it is the density per housing unit that explains local variation in

neighborhood may be caused by the bad quality of the housing stock and may require a different housing policy rather than only a medical response.

Proponents of a neighborhood-based approach to health care argue that, in opposition to the more sectoral approach pursued by national state bureaucracies, 'local care teams' can mobilize local social knowledge to pursue a more holistic approach in which a focus on physical health is combined with attention to general well-being, as well as socio-spatial needs, such as well-ventilated housing. For elderly citizens, for example, problems of loneliness due to weaker social networks may lead to a decrease in well-being, but also to a higher risk that medical problems are not detected on time. Turning the post-COVID-19 city into an 'equally healthy' city requires urban planners to pay attention to health inequalities. One way of doing this is by putting health facilities central in the spatial programming for neighborhoods in urban renewal. In this way, neighborhood health care centers can provide new forms of socio-spatial centrality and create an equalizing version of the 15-minute city.

Conclusion

For us, one of the essential questions the pandemic has raised (again) to urban researchers and urban policy makers is how the city could act as an 'equalizer'. How could we appreciate (and move beyond) the city as a platform for survival and social mobility for disadvantaged groups?

Apart from a more genuine involvement of all space-users in urban decision-making as well as civil society organizations that give voice to the voiceless (see also Volume 2, Chapter Sixteen), it seems important to look for new methods in urban (planning) policy to leave the 'normative' point of view when planning for the 'vulnerable city'. Indeed, today urban (planning) policy is still too much a reflection of the profile of the often 'white', middle-class (and male) urban planner or policy maker. Hence, it is important to understand that the own experience (of the planner or policy maker) is not universal, but in many ways normative and privileged. The introduction of new methods, such as an ethnographic approach to space or participatory action research, to overcome this gap are indispensable.

Lastly, it is important to acknowledge that the intervention of urban policy makers and planners in urban space is not (only) a scientific exercise, but above all a matter of political choices. In that regard, it is important to remain vigilant. History learns that 'health crises' have often been (mis)used by urban policy makers to serve other agendas than public health. Global history is replete with incidences of low-income groups or minority groups being evicted from neighborhoods with (potentially) high real estate value under the pretext of health care and hygiene (Beeckmans, 2016). As a result, all too often health care measures have (un)consciously led to new patterns of exclusion and socio-spatial segregation. By addressing the socio-spatial needs of the most vulnerable groups in COVID-19 times, we hope the COVID-19 city will find inspiration to break with this tradition.

References

Beeckmans, L. (2016) 'A toponymy of segregation: the "neutral zones" of Dakar, Dar Es Salaam and Kinshasa', in L. Bigon (ed) *Place Names in Africa: Colonial Urban Legacies, Entangled Histories*. Switzerland: Springer, pp 105–22.

Beeckmans, L. (2020a) 'A plea for greater diversity in urban redevelopment', in S. De Caigny (ed) *When Attitudes Take Form. Flanders Architectural Review N°14*. Antwerp: Flanders Architecture Institute, pp 129–36.

Beeckmans, L. (2020b) 'Hoe laten we COVID-19 onze steden hertekenen?' *Knack*, April 22. Retrieved from: www.knack. be/nieuws/belgie/hoe-laten-we-COVID-19-onze-steden-hertekenen/article-opinion-1591235.html

Boie, G. (2020) 'De stad hertekenen, nu kan het'. *De Standaard*, April 15. Retrieved from: www.standaard.be/cnt/dmf20200414_04922610

Braekman, K. and Hofman, A. (2020) 'Vastgoed boomt: corona maakt huis met tuin en appartement aan de kust populair'. *VRT News*, September 3. Retrieved from: www.vrt.be/vrtnws/nl/2020/09/02/vastgoed-corona-maakt-huis-met-tuin-en-belgische-kust-populair/

Bruzz (2020) 'Oversterfte door COVID: Vooral in Brussel wordt lage sociale klasse het hardst getroffen'. *Bruzz*, October 10. Retrieved from: www.bruzz.be/samenleving/oversterfte-door-covid-vooral-brussel-wordt-lage-sociale-klasse-het-hardst-getroffen

Colson, J. (2020) 'Pleit niet voor een universeel basisinkomen, maar voor universele huisvesting'. *Knack*, April 17. Retrieved from: www.knack.be/nieuws/belgie/pleit-niet-voor-een-universeel-basisinkomen-maar-voor-universele-huisvesting/article-opinion-1589323.html

De Decker, P. (2020) 'Bouwen aan een gemengde wijk'. *De Standaard*, June 17. Retrieved from: www.standaard.be/cnt/dmf20200616_04992959?fbclid=IwAR0B015r3q6a1nIw7k1BX05Qy0fGqJfRyfQPGWOiyz0ZSrAfpWa2WXsEP04

Delepeleire, Y. (2020, May 23) 'Jongeren eisen het recht op om rond te hangen'. *De Standaard*. Retrieved from: www.standaard.be/cnt/dmf20200522_04968732

De Smet, D. (2020) 'Twee tot drie keer meer covid-19-overlijdens bij armste inkomens'. *De Standaard*, October 14. Retrieved from: www.standaard.be/cnt/dmf20201014_94179788

Gehl, J. (2020) *Public Space, Public Life & COVID-19*. Retrieved from: covid19.gehlpeople.com

Gehl, J. and Svarre, B. (2013) *How to Study Public Life*. Copenhagen: Island Press/Center for Resource Economics.

Ghys, T. and Oosterlynck, S. (2017) *Sociale innovaties bekeken vanuit structurele armoedebestrijding: case Wijkgezondheidscentra*. Antwerp: Vlaams Armoedesteunpunt.

Goossens, C., Oosterlynck, S. and Bradt, L. (2019) 'Livable streets? Green gentrification and the displacement of longtime residents in Ghent, Belgium'. *Urban Geography*, DOI: 10.1080/02723638.2019.1686307

Nieuwsblad (2020) 'Mag overheid verbieden om in tijden van lockdown naar tweede verblijf aan de kust te gaan?' *Nieuwsblad*, May 13. Retrieved from: www.nieuwsblad.be/cnt/dmf20200513_04957243

Renson, I. (2020) 'Worden de steden winnaars of verliezers van corona?' *De Standaard*, May 9. Retrieved from: www.standaard.be/cnt/dmf20200508_04951870

Rogers, A. (2020) 'How does a virus spread in cities? It's a problem of scale'. *Wired*, May 5. Retrieved from: www.wired.com/story/how-does-a-virus-spread-in-cities-its-a-problem-of-scale

Van Acker, M. (2020) ''t Stad als vaccin, onze buurt als medicijn'. *Gazet Van Antwerpen*, April 15. Retrieved from: www.gva.be/cnt/dmf20200415_04923077

VRP (2020) 'PostCoronaTalks: Hoe maken we de stad gezond?' *Vereniging Ruimte en Planning (VRP)*. Retrieved from: www.vrp.be/activiteit/postcoronatalks

(Goldstein, 2010) of a health crisis provided police forces with exceptional powers, similar to those given during times of terrorist threat.

In the securitization logic of the lockdown, the police increasingly focused on maintaining order in public space and keeping 'everyone in their "proper" place in the seemingly natural order of things' (Dikeç, 2005: 174). Hayward (2012) uses the metaphor of 'container spaces' while discussing police strategies like 'kettling' – a means of containing and enclosing protesters into a designated perimeter. The police became managers of public space, moving populations to designed places, like board game players moving pieces around. As Rancière (2001: 8) cynically noted ' "Move along! There is nothing to see here!" The police says that there is nothing to see on a road, that there is nothing to do but move along. It asserts that the space of circulating is nothing other than the space of circulation.'

The displacement of vulnerable populations reveals an aspect of police work that is less related to crime control, and more to a kind of theater or performance: 'the policing of undesirable bodies and practices is not simply about quantitative crime reduction, but conducted through qualitative, embodied performance' (Cook and Whowell, 2011: 610). Police officers are guards of the moral dimensions of *publicness*, in which vulnerable populations are barred from exceeding what Brighenti (2010: 47) called 'the upper threshold of correct visibility'. Atkinson (2003: 1838), in a different, but nonetheless relevant context, coins the term 'domestication by cappuccino', referring to 'a public realm strategy by the local authority and police which supports the removal of those people who tarnish its image'.

During the first weeks of the COVID-19 lockdown in Brussels (March to early June 2020), both securitization and displacement were easily observable. While public spaces instantly became desolate – even emptier than after the terrorist attacks of March 22, 2016 – groups such as the homeless and undocumented migrants had no option than to stay in these empty public spaces, accompanied only by police patrols. The co-presence of homeless and police officers did not occur without conflict: outreach workers signaled many cases of homeless and undocumented migrants being questioned, given fines, and of being chased away for simply sitting for a short period of time on a bench or in a park.

This chapter presents some early findings from ongoing research (by the first author) on refugees, asylum-seekers, undocumented migrants, and homeless (hereafter 'vulnerable groups') in public spaces during the COVID-19 crisis. During the months of March, April, and May, 30 interviews were undertaken with frontline practitioners such as social assistants, social workers, teachers in basic education, outreach workers, and youth workers. Instead of talking directly with vulnerable individuals, which we felt would be unethical and contribute to higher levels of stress in their already dire circumstances, we relied on practitioners with a good inside knowledge of the everyday conflicts between police and vulnerable populations. Our initial findings show how the pandemic impacted the lives of vulnerable urban populations, and how the consequences of the increased policing of public spaces adversely affects the lives of these populations.

Vulnerable groups in public space

In the first weeks of the lockdown, many services closed their doors. For instance, Benny, an asylum lawyer, explained how the national reception center for asylum-seekers *Dienst Vreemdelingenzaken* (DVZ; literally translated 'Office for Foreigner Affairs') had closed its doors. As a result, some newcomers were not granted their right to request asylum and also missed out on the orientation service – which would have included referral to legal advice – usually provided at DVZ. Moreover, many other basic services such as day and night shelters closed instantly. According to Yamina, a youth worker volunteering in food distribution for the homeless, "The shelter has converted its restaurant to a sleeping room, but during the day [homeless people] are forced to go into the street."

Due to the lack of accessible and safe spaces elsewhere, many vulnerable populations were increasingly dependent on public spaces. Nelly, a social assistant engaged in food distribution, feared for those who for various reasons, would be unable to find her organization and end up living on the streets. She was afraid "that they feel very lonely, more excluded than usual, and they currently have a life where they wander around and are chased away everywhere". Even her own organization chased people away after they got their meals, because otherwise neighbors complained and called the police. Mohamed, a social worker in an asylum institution for unaccompanied minors, argued that the closure of DVZ forced asylum-seekers to the Maximiliaan Park in Brussels where *impromptu* food and clothes distribution was organized by citizen initiatives and NGOs. He explained that "temporary housing should have been provided for these groups that live on the street, if necessary, in the park, in tents, to give these people masks, hand sanitizer. It is a rather large group". Instead, the groups were chased away by the police, who justified their actions by referring to the ban on public gathering.

Some groups reacted without a sense of urgency, said youth worker Jonas. "They are hanging out, giving a hand, a kiss, a handclap, they play a match of soccer, all very cosy". He called it "youthful hubris". Phillip similarly noted, that particularly in the first few weeks, the homeless and undocumented migrants he worked with were in a "party mode": "You bombard them with calamity messages, but they feel they cannot prevent that calamity. They're a bit like a brass band on the Titanic." Other groups were more nervous. As one outreach worker put it: "You feel the tension, those young people and young adults hanging out, who have way too much time […] it doesn't take much for situations to go wrong."

Both the sanitary and security measures had a profound impact on the life of vulnerable groups. The measures fundamentally changed the way these groups used and interacted with public space. Their already precarious condition was magnified by these changes, which as we show later, were compounded by their daily, and problematic, experiences with the Brussels police.

Policing the pandemic

'Everybody has to move, you can't stand still. Homeless people are tired of being constantly on the move, you can't sit on a bench anymore.'

'They're constantly being addressed on the street by the police [...] Yesterday at the food distribution a young man came to pick up food and fill his bag, and he asks: "What should I say to the police if they stop me?" I say, "But they're not going to stop you." "Yes, I was stopped on my way here, and they asked me what you were doing on the street." That scared me.'

In the early days of the lockdown, this was how Phillip and Nelly, respectively, commented on the police action in public space. Similarly, Mieke, a social assistant, recounted that it was forbidden to "walk the streets with more than two people, we have to be very cautious", while Nora, a youth worker, further predicted that "if they continue to be tough on this ban, things will explode. There are people who just live in very small houses or apartments, right?" Jonas, an outreach worker, added that this type of intensive policing came on top of the already strained relationship between certain migrant groups and the police. Benny commented that, "The mayor has announced that police action will be strict and you know that also before the crisis there was much racism in the police force. I can imagine that some of these officers now see an opportunity for payback time." Phillip agreed: "There certainly is abuse of power [...], there is a small percentage [of police officers] who are having a good time."

In retrospect, some actors, such as the state and its security forces, may be inclined to frame their actions during the lockdown as *force majeure* and the improvisation of measures in an exceptional crisis. But it remains all the more noteworthy that the way the sanitary and security crisis was handled by these actors has provided their critics with more examples of the familiar practices which characterize the biased enforcement of public order.

References

Atkinson, R. (2003) 'Domestication by cappuccino or a revenge on urban space? Control and empowerment in the management of public spaces'. *Urban Studies*, 40(9): 1829–43.

Brighenti, A.M. (2010) *Visibility in Social Theory and Social Research.* New York: Palgrave Macmillan.

Cook, I.R. and Whowell, M. (2011) 'Visibility and the policing of public space'. *Geography Compass*, 8: 610–22.

Dikeç, M. (2005)'. 'Space, politics, and the political'. *Environment and Planning D: Society and Space*, 23: 171–88.

Goedgebeur, H. (2020) '235 klachten over corona-interventies van politie: "Onterecht, slecht behandeld of passieve houding".' *vrtnws.be.* www.vrt.be/vrtnws/nl/2020/08/06/235-klachten-over-corona-interventies-van-politie/

Goldstein, D.M. (2010) 'Toward a critical anthropology of security'. *Current Anthropology*, 51(4): 487–517.

Hayward, K. (2012) 'Five spaces of cultural criminology'. *British Journal of Criminology*, 52: 441–62.

Rancière, J. (2001) 'Ten theses on politics'. Translated by D. Panagia and R. Bowlby. *Theory & Event*, 5(3): 1–16.

SIX

Parks in a Pandemic: Attachments, Absences, and Exclusions

Julian Dobson

Introduction

Neglected and underfunded after a decade of austerity, urban parks in the UK were thrust into the limelight by the COVID-19 pandemic. During the spring lockdown, they were among the few public spaces that remained open and accessible. The management of the pandemic was marked by changes in rules about what could or could not be done outside.

The imposition of rules on the use of public space, and public reactions to them, highlight both the value and the contested character of urban green spaces (see also Chapters Eight and Nine, this volume). Focusing on Sheffield, a post-industrial city in northern England, this chapter considers how space can be understood through personal and community attachments to places, and public and political responses to COVID-19. It explores how the visibility and invisibility of different publics engaged in everyday leisure activities exposes underlying inequalities.

It begins by outlining parks' historic background as appreciated but depreciating urban assets and briefly charts the course of the lockdown as it affected public space in England.

It then examines the experience of lockdown in four urban green spaces, first in terms of attachments to place and then in terms of absences. It discusses whether absences are, or could become, exclusions, curtailing the value of green spaces as genuinely public. Finally it reflects on the future of urban parks in the light of current policy directions.

Lockdown

To understand UK parks' current position and the importance of their role during the lockdown, we need to rewind the clock 40 years. The dismantling of the post-war welfare state saw a race to the bottom in terms of maintenance and management as municipalities were compelled to put greenspace services out to competitive tender to cut costs and – ostensibly – reduce the burden on local taxpayers (see also Chapter Seven, this volume).

This in turn prompted a rediscovery of the value of parks and a decade of reinvestment at the turn of the millennium. The current of policy shifted again after 2010 when Britain's Coalition government introduced a decade of austerity, with the ax falling particularly heavily on local councils, which own and manage most parks. By 2017 a parliamentary investigation declared England's parks to be at 'a tipping point of decline' (House of Commons Communities and Local Government Committee, 2017). Against this backdrop, landscape academics and managers were initially relieved when the importance of parks was explicitly recognized in the first stages of the lockdown. The nationwide lockdown announced on March 23 permitted a small range of exceptions: shopping for necessities, medical emergencies, helping a vulnerable person, travel for essential work – and one form of exercise a day. For such exercise, parks would stay open. But only two people could be together in public unless they were from the same household.

Not all parks stayed open. As pubs, shops, and restaurants pulled down security shutters, citizens flocked to urban open spaces – and some park managers responded by locking them, warning that the overcrowding was unsafe. London's original public park, Victoria Park in Tower Hamlets, was one of the first to bolt its gates. Middlesbrough's Albert Park was another prominent closure.

On April 18 Secretary of State for Housing and Communities Robert Jenrick, responding to press questions, insisted parks should remain open so people could get fresh air and exercise. As restrictions were relaxed, so was access to green space. On May 10 the prime minister lifted the 'once a day' rule on outdoor exercise. People could now spend time outdoors as long as they complied with social distancing advice and did not meet more than one person at a time from outside their household. On June 1 the restrictions were eased again, allowing up to six people to meet outdoors.

The new advice recognized the reduced risk of infection in outdoor environments. But it also appeared that the government had taken note of the extensive evidence of their value for health and well-being, both within the UK (Dobson et al, 2019) and internationally (World Health Organization, 2016).

Attachments

The notion of place attachment is rooted in studies of what Low and Altman (1992) describe as 'the unique emotional experiences and bond of people with places'. These can include notions of the sacred and special, but also of the mundane and familiar. Gieryn (2000) describes places as 'doubly constructed: most are built or in some way physically carved out. They are also interpreted, narrated, perceived, felt, understood, and imagined'.

These connections are not only individual. Manzo and Perkins (2006) note that 'emotional connection is at the core of a sense of community'. Belonging exists in relation to the materiality of places as well as to social groups, and social groups shape the materiality of places. The presence or absence of particular groups is echoed in landscape.

was reduced to minimal intervention by paid professionals, with an emphasis on safety rather than sociability.

Absences were particularly evident in Heeley Park. Carved out of derelict space between housing estates on one of Sheffield's many steep hillsides, it is the city's largest community-owned park. In 1996 the land was transferred from the municipality to Heeley Trust, a community organization that has labored to address issues of poverty and disadvantage.

At the heart of Heeley Park is a 'crow's nest' wooden sculpture that acts as both a viewpoint and a youth shelter, a place to hang out or to watch the sunset. There is a children's playground (more imaginatively designed than most), spaces for picnics and sports, wooded areas, and cycleways. More importantly, this is a place where the local community have a say in what goes on, and can get involved in events and festivals.

During the lockdown the park was almost deserted – the occasional desultory dog walker, a couple of youths on bikes. The public space had become an empty container, almost devoid of its public. Lockdown had defamiliarized the space. The views remained, but the viewers were missing.

There were other absences almost everywhere. Those who could not get out without the support of a carer or health care professional – people with learning or physical disabilities, for example – were largely missing. Those who had to 'shield' because of their vulnerability to COVID-19 were confined to their homes. Older people disappeared from some of the more popular parks as groups of young people occupied the space.

Exclusions

The word 'absence' suggests something missing, but it also misses something. The absences connected with COVID-19 were not voluntary. Green spaces were not only valued and appreciated during lockdown: they were regulated and policed. The process of regulation was also one of exclusion.

Manzo and Perkins (2006: 337) describe place attachment as 'a dynamic and dialectic process that includes both a positive and a "shadow" side, as attachments can also entrap or create territorial conflicts'. This raises the question of whose attachments are perceived to matter.

In the early stages of lockdown this prescriptive and proscriptive approach to green spaces, and to the emotional connections associated with those uses, was especially evident in Sheffield's Botanical Gardens. The gardens are the city's horticultural jewel, laid out by the renowned Victorian landscaper Robert Marnock. The elegant glasshouses with their collections of tropical and desert plants were closed. So too was the popular cafe, the necessary public toilets, and the classroom where gardening experts give well-attended talks. On the entrance gates were notices headlined STAY AT HOME in red lettering. Benches were taped over to stop anyone sitting on them (Figure 6.1).

Figure 6.1: Taped over benches at Sheffield's Botanical Gardens

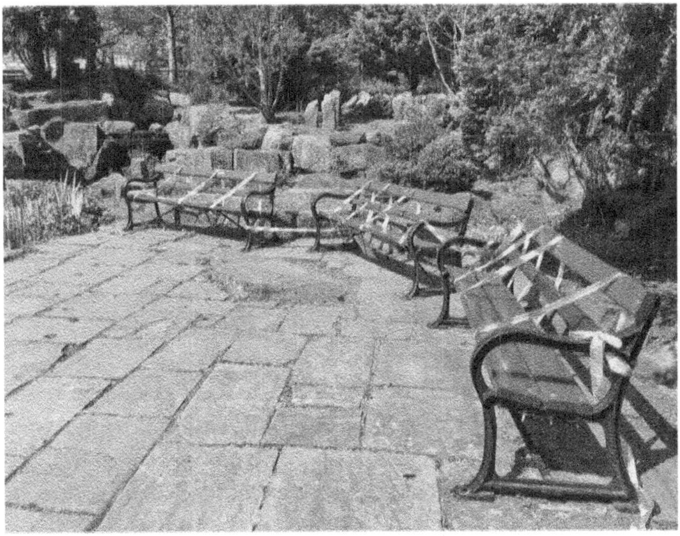

Source: Julian Dobson

In this phase of lockdown the public park became a site of enforced mobility, a conveyor belt of citizens engaged in mutual policing of unwritten 'no loitering' regulations. Little thought was given to those who cannot use a park without being able to stop and sit for a moment, or visit a public toilet if needed. While parks filled up during weeks of sunshine, those with disabilities or mobility difficulties became invisible. The consequences were profoundly unequal, impacting most severely on the already vulnerable.

Futures

The unanticipated prominence of parks during the pandemic led to a redoubling by greenspace professionals of evidence-gathering, lobbying, and argument in favor of renewed investment in green spaces. But in a policy context in which the government's slogan for post-pandemic recovery is 'build, build, build' there is a growing risk that the need to support and restore the place attachments of more vulnerable people will be overlooked.

In August 2020 the UK government published a planning white paper (Ministry of Housing, Communities and Local Government, 2020) which purported to provide a 'fast-track to beauty'. Its deregulatory thrust implied that inclusive or democratic approaches to planning are a hindrance to high-quality places rather than their guardian. At a time when urban green spaces have been underfunded and municipal costs are escalating, the planning white paper has aggravated the threats of sale, excessive commercialization, and inappropriate development.

Yet there remains an opportunity to rediscover the value of parks as health-giving, inclusive, and democratizing – and as spaces where all social groups can find new attachments to the natural world. COVID-19 has shown the persistence of privilege, even in spaces that are apparently equitable. In considering how we can make the best of green spaces in a post-pandemic world, we must extend the benefits they offer to publics who often remain invisible and who have been further excluded as a consequence of the events of 2020.

Note

While the evidence cited on p 57 was the product of collaborative work with colleagues at the University of Sheffield and Sheffield Hallam University, the views expressed are the author's own.

References

Dobson, J., Harris, C., Eadson, W. and Gore, T. (2019) *Space to Thrive: A Rapid Evidence Review of the Benefits of Parks and Green Spaces for People and Communities.* London: The National Lottery Heritage Fund and The National Lottery Community Fund.

Gieryn, T.F. (2000) 'A space for place in sociology'. *Annual Review of Sociology*, 26: 463–96.

House of Commons Communities and Local Government Committee (2017) *Public parks: Seventh report of session 2016–17.* https://publications.parliament.uk/pa/cm201617/cmselect/cmcomloc/45/45.pdf

Ingold, T. (2011) *Being Alive: Essays on Movement, Knowledge and Description.* Abingdon: Routledge.

Low, S. and Altman, I. (1992) 'Place attachment', in I. Altman and S. Low (eds) *Place Attachment.* New York: Springer, pp 1–12.

Manzo, L. and Perkins, D. (2006) 'Finding common ground: the importance of place attachment to community participation and planning'. *Journal of Planning Literature*, 20(4): 335–50.

Ministry of Housing, Communities and Local Government (2020) Planning for the Future. https://assets.publishing.service.gov.uk/government/uploads/system/uploads/attachment_data/file/907647/MHCLG-Planning-Consultation.pdf

World Health Organization (2016) Urban green spaces and health: A review of evidence. www.euro.who.int/__data/assets/pdf_file/0005/321971/Urban-green-spaces-and-health-review-evidence.pdf?ua=1

with increasingly vitriolic responses, being held accountable for the spread of the virus and the UK's bourgeoning death toll. The term 'covidiots' quickly infiltrated the lexicon of public discourse amid condemnation of those seen to be using parks, beaches, and other public spaces. The (mis)use of public space had, it seems, become one of the key battlegrounds of cities under lockdown.

That transgression of the 'stay home' imperative, framed around the supposed failure of the individual, is perhaps unsurprising when considered as an expression of neoliberal discourse on individual responsibility, and regulation of public space. The individualistic narrative that emerged during the COVID-19 lockdown appears to be a logical extension of social, spatial, and political transformations undertaken under the banner of neoliberalism. However, the conventional understanding of lockdown restrictions and non-compliance elides, inter alia, an understanding of the inter and intra urban inequalities. In this chapter, I begin by briefly sketching out the way in which the 'lockdown', and individualistic narratives depicting those who (mis)use public space as 'covidiots', exacerbates spatial inequalities which are built into the fabric of densely populated cities. I will conclude by framing this by reflecting on the (im)possibility of compliance with lockdown measures in the (neoliberal) city.

Public space, urban inequality, and the lockdown

In the initial phase of lockdown in the UK, beginning on March 23, the issue of public space became increasingly prominent in public discourse. In particular, pictures of busy parks, beaches, and other public spaces were read, in the public imagination at least, as evidence of lockdown transgression and moral failure. Through this lens, the 'selfishness' of those who (mis)use public space during lockdown and 'recklessly' endanger the lives of others punctures the solidarity expressed by those who stay home. As such, the term 'covidiot' quickly established itself in the lexicon of public discourse, to describe those suspected of lockdown transgression. Local newspapers headlines proclaimed that 'Londoners bask in park sunshine despite Boris Johnson begging people to stay home during COVID-19 lockdown' (Brewis, 2020), illustrating the degree to which the issue of lockdown compliance had become individualized, with the government – apparently – lacking powers of enforcement beyond appealing to individual 'common-sense'. Further, the widespread use of #selfishpricks, often tweeted in response to pictures of busy public spaces, to decry the 'selfishness' of individuals using public space during the lockdown further reinforces the extent to which lockdown compliance had become an issue of individual moral responsibility.

An unambiguous narrative had, therefore, emerged. A narrative which foregrounds individual (mis)use of public space and non-compliance with lockdown restrictions as opposed to the nature, and enforcement, of the lockdown itself. What this narrative elides, however, is the extent to which the battle for public space in cities under lockdown is consistent with the spatial inequalities of the neoliberal city. Indeed, the rise of neoliberalism has been concomitant with an increasing (re)regulation, privatization, and commodification of public space (Smith and Low, 2006). Some scholars have situated this shift within broader ideological assault, invoking an increasingly revanchist, or punitive, political assault on minoritized groups (for example, Smith, 1996; MacLeod, 2002; Lawton, 2018). As MacLeod (2002: 603) states, the neoliberal urban form is 'increasingly choreographed through control over and purification of urban (public) space'. It is within this context, within the 'trenchant reregulation and redaction of public space' (Smith and Low, 2006: 1), that we must situate the COVID-19 lockdown in the UK (see also Chapter Twelve, this volume).

At the most basic level, the continued use of public spaces, such as parks, amid the lockdown is a reflection of the socio-spatial fabric of cities themselves. It will come as a surprise to little that those living in densely populated cities have less access to private outdoor space when compared with their rural or suburban counterparts. Hence, Andrew Smith (2020: 3) argues that '(parks) [are] fundamental pieces of green infrastructure that make our cities more sustainable and liveable'. In focusing, however, on the behavior of the individual using the 'covidiot' mantra, this elides the systemic factors which can drive (mis)use of public space, such as a lack of alternative green spaces out with local parks. It seems, therefore, that the issue of compliance with lockdown measures is not the failure of the individual, but rather failure by design – especially given the dubious logic of the covidiot narrative which suggests that the mere use of parks as tantamount to lockdown transgression. Access and availability of public and private outdoors space(s) is not politically neutral nor coincidental. It seems that by shaming those who have little choice but to 'congregate' in public spaces refracts the dominant spatial inequity of lockdown itself, insofar as this can be connected to access and availability of private outdoor spaces.

It is within this context that attention must (re)turn to issues of compliance, and the 'policing' of lockdown restrictions on public space. Issues relating to lockdown compliance have been policed, principally, by creating narrative forms – such as the covidiot narrative – which encourage compliance by 'shaming' those who fail to comply as well as encouraging the public to become informants within their communities. UK Health Secretary Matt Hancock, for example, has claimed that he would 'snitch' on his neighbor for lockdown non-compliance, and added that it is the public's responsibility to avoid 'tougher' lockdown measures by complying with restrictions (Owen, 2020). This message seemingly resonated with a frightened public. In Humberside, for example, the local police received around 900 calls per day about lockdown non-compliance, which prompted the police force to brand the restrictions themselves as 'woolly' and open to interpretation (ITV, 2020).

This reinforces the surveillance and regulation of public space which embodies neoliberal urbanism by encouraging the public themselves to become participants in it.

In addition to this, police responses to the lockdown imperative further contours the developments of urban neoliberalism, particularly as this pertains to increasing regulation of public spaces such as parks. Indeed, police powers of enforcement during the lockdown mark a continuation of revanchist police practice which permeates urban neoliberalism, with controversial tactics such as stop-and-search and powers of dispersal used to curtail certain uses and users of public spaces. Indeed, by May 25, police had issued 15,552 fixed penalty notices for lockdown non-compliance, while aiming to 'ensure voluntary compliance' with measures in England (National Police Chiefs' Council (NPCC), 2020). This, of course, resembles what Setha Low (2015: 154) articulates, in the context of the US, as the neoliberal model of public space which relies on 'the militarisation and penetration of surveillance and policing apparatus to remove "undesirables".' The COVID-19 lockdown has, therefore, exacerbated already established models of neoliberal urban governance and police practice which constricts the use and availability of public space, particularly in dense urban centers and gentrifying areas.

In any case, it is clear that focusing on 'individual responsibility' elides the way in which lockdown enforcement has been undermined by an assemblage of socio-spatial inequality and government (in)action. To be clear, this is not to suggest that individuals cannot act irresponsibly. Rather, this suggests that focusing on personal responsibility does not account for the systemic nature of lockdown compliance. Further, the covidiot narrative cannot simply be read as reactionary impulse against those visibly using public space despite the 'stay home' guidance. Rather, this reflects the dominance of neoliberalism within the lexicon of public discourse and government policy. Demonstrating, as Harvey (2007) argues, that neoliberalism has infiltrated our common-sense understanding of the world.

restrictions placed upon residents have exacerbated existing discourse(s), tensions, and inequalities within the neoliberal city. It is clear, therefore, that the individualistic narrative that has been mainstreamed throughout the initial peak of COVID-19 in the UK is an insufficient explanation of issues of lockdown compliance in the UK. To begin, it is necessary to consider the situated, and context-specific, nature of lockdown transgressions. It should come as little surprise, therefore, that when we consider the way in which public space has contracted in the neoliberal era, that access and availability of public spaces should be foregrounded during the lockdown. The individualistic mantra that has emerged in reaction to the 'selfishness' of those who use public space during the lockdown elides a more meaningful comment on systemic nature of 'lockdown' transgression and inequity in their application. Second, in addition to the socio-spatial nature of the neoliberal city, I have also demonstrated the ideological nature of the 'covidiot' narrative which accepts, uncritically, neoliberal conceptions of individual responsibility and in doing so, pathologizes individual (mis)uses of space as opposed to commenting on the inherently politicized nature of such (mis)use.

References

Brewis, H. (2020) 'Londoners bask in park sunshine despite Boris Johnson begging people to stay home during COVID-19 lockdown'. *London Evening Standard*, April 5. Retrieved from: www.standard.co.uk/

Hackworth, J. and Moriah, A. (2006) 'Neoliberalism, contingency and urban policy: the case of social housing in Ontario'. *International Journal of Urban and Regional Research*, 30(3): 510–27.

Harvey, D. (2007) *A Brief Introduction to Neoliberalism*. Oxford: Oxford University Press.

ITV News (2020, July 10) 'Humberside Police received 900 complaints a day during lockdown about people breaking social distancing rules'. *ITV News*. Retrieved from: www.itv.com/news/calendar/2020-07-10/humberside-police-received-900-complaints-a-day-during-lockdown-about-people-breaking-social-distancing-rules

Lawton, P. (2018) 'Situating revanchism in the contemporary city'. *City*, 22 (5–6): 867–74.

Low, S. (2015) 'Public space and the public sphere: the legacy of Neil Smith'. *Antipode*, 49(1): 153–70.

MacLeod, G. (2002) 'From urban entrepreneurialism to a "revanchist city"? On the spatial injustices of Glasgow's Renaissance'. *Antipode*, 34(3): 602–24.

McGregor, S. (2008) 'Neoliberalism and health care'. *International Journal of Consumer Studies*, 25(2): 82–9.

National Police Chiefs' Council (NPCC) (2020) Statistical update on number of lockdown fines given by police. Retrieved from: https://news.npcc.police.uk/releases/statistical-update-on-number-of-lockdown-fines-given-by-police

Owen, B. (2020) 'Matt Hancock said he would snitch on his own neighbour for not isolating'. *Metro*, September 20. Retrieved from: https://metro.co.uk/2020/09/20/matt-hancock-said-he-would-snitch-on-his-own-neighbour-for-not-self-isolating-13298144/

Smith, A. (2020) 'Sustaining municipal parks in an era of neoliberal austerity: the contested commercialisation of Gunnersbury Park'. *Environment and Planning A: Economy and Space*, https://doi.org/10.1177/0308518X20951814

Smith, N. (1996) *The New Urban Frontier: Gentrification and the Revanchist City*. London: Routledge.

Smith, N. and Low, S. (2006) 'Introduction: The imperative of public space', in S. Low and N. Smith (eds) *The Politics of Public Space*. London: Routledge.

Srnieck, N. and Williams, A. (2015) *Inventing the Future: Postcaptialism and a World Without Work*. London: Verso.

EIGHT

A Place for Life: Striving Towards Accessible and Equitable Public Spaces for Times of Crisis and Beyond

Anaid Yerena and Rubén Casas

Introduction

In this chapter, we take from definitions of public open space offered by Montejano-Castillo and Moreno-Villanueva (2016) and Jian et al (2020) to say that public open space, which includes streets, sidewalks, parks, plazas, and playgrounds, and other spaces funded by and for general public use, is fundamental to the production of just cities which promote health and wellness among residents, especially during public health crises.

The availability and quality of public open space correlate with increased physical and mental health, to the vitality of community life, and to the strength and resilience of the social fabric (Krellenberg et al, 2014; Chen et. al, 2016; Jennings et al, 2016). Klinenberg (2015) argues that 'social infrastructure', which includes open public spaces, is essential to the survival of more people in times of crisis as it is this infrastructure that line with our experiences of the COVID-19 pandemic. We have abundant scientific evidence that access to the outdoors in times of crisis results in better physical and mental health (The Trust for Public Land, 2020).

Crisis in the unequitable city

One way of explaining the uneven experience of the COVID-19 pandemic is by applying Fainstein's (2009) sense that most cities are now run by/for capital, which has reduced the amount of public investment that results in more equitable infrastructure. Given these neoliberal orientations, open public space that is not generating wealth is not prioritized, and the little public monies that do exist go towards creating further comfort for the already well-off. Cash-strapped cities that are focused on making themselves more attractive to external capital are likely to see many of their residents suffer more acutely during pandemics as they realize that they lack ample open public space, and that which they do have is ill-maintained or poorly equipped to accommodate many visitors seeking to maintain distance.

Even those cities which do count on ample open space do not always invest in creating the necessary access to it. In many cases, parks are at a reasonable distance if traveling by car but not on foot or if assisted by a mobility device; some are not served by transit. In certain neighborhoods a lack of sidewalks, crosswalks, and adequate lighting make the trip to the park treacherous (Boone et al, 2009). Often, areas lacking parks are also lacking this essential infrastructure, making the disparities in open public space especially acute. Renters or people living in small units are the ones most impacted (Wolch et al, 2005).

These common realities do not just occur on their own, rather they are created. Edward Soja's concept of spatial justice, an idea concerned with showing 'how the spaces in which we live are socially produced' (2013: 7), reminds us of this disconnect. Spatial justice also presents a viable way of redressing injustice in the modern city by centering those most impacted by injustice, allowing them a greater say in how we remake the city to better serve the needs of all.

In the wake of the COVID-19 pandemic, we can plan for future parks and open public spaces that prove resilient and which in turn build resilience within the open space infrastructure that already exists (see also Chapter Nine, this volume). During COVID-19, some cities have demonstrated dexterity by reopening their roads to more multimodal use and by permitting public and private proposals that reclaim parking for greater use. We argue that these reclamations of space should be adopted permanently because they represent greater, more equitable use of public space in general.

Recommendations

We offer several recommendations on how cities can recognize the vital role of parks in times of crisis; we have organized these into four groups.

First, fund open spaces with public monies. In the US, '[a]round 30% of park funding comes from commercial sources' (Barker and Smith, 2020). In an era of declining tax revenues and privatization, many cities have to seek out grants to fund new parks and maintain existing ones (Holifield and Williams, 2014). While grant funding is not to be disparaged, it does create further inequity since some cities count with the staff and expertise to secure grants while others do not (Wolch et al, 2005). Cities must earmark public funds and lobby state and federal legislators to ensure that adequate funding structures exist so that all residents are served by parks. Since public open spaces depend on stable, predictable public funding, identifying new funding sources is paramount to their existence.

Second, reclaim underused public space, for example by reopening streets to pedestrian-only use (see also Chapter Sixteen, this volume). The amount of land and money our cities devote to cars is unconscionable; reclaiming strategic portions of these resources will shift priority towards greater access for people and sustainability and redress this imbalance. Reclaiming some of this land for pedestrians and mobility devices (for example wheelchairs, strollers, bikes) requires planning and strategizing. Local authorities already control this land; its upkeep and operation are mostly governed by the city's transportation plans. Priority areas for this approach include streets adjacent to parks, main streets, alleys, and streets that divide parks. Paramount to proper implementation is considering adjacent uses and destinations, so these pedestrianized thoroughfares actually meet transportation needs.

Other options are to repurpose public schools' outdoor areas as well as the outdoor areas of civic and government buildings, and those in public college and university campuses. Most public schools have some outdoor space, these spaces' after-hours use usually remain unused and closed to the public. Determining guidelines for how to share these outdoor areas with the rest of the community is the first priority. Public school districts have oversight of these spaces and will need to coordinate with local park authorities to identify and pre-empt potential conflicts. Many public institutions have well-maintained, attractive green spaces, plazas, and quads that can be made more accessible to more people. Often, these spaces are reserved for those who work or study there, or those needing to pay a bill or make an inquiry. Again, these spaces often sit unused in the evenings and weekends. We argue these spaces should be welcoming to residents at large, in particular within urban campuses. Cities can work with facilities and grounds managers to activate these spaces to serve residents, even when the buildings themselves are closed. Lastly, streets (as greenways) between parks and green spaces need to be revamped. As cities around the US implement complete streets in order to serve the needs of more people needing to get outdoors near their homes, we argue these expanded uses can be adopted and developed upon to ensure that these equitable uses of existing underused public infrastructure remain in less dire times. Complete streets rely on building a network of streets that connect you to points of interest; parks and open public spaces are clear examples of points of interest; complete streets are achievable by expanding the uses of existing streets.

Third, manage facilities to optimize capacity, maintain, and program recreation facilities in culturally relevant ways. Many parks and green spaces are underutilized simply because they are non-managed (Boone et al, 2009); municipal corporations that care for these spaces play a key role in their programming. Often, parks that are meant to serve low-income neighborhoods suffer the most neglect. Seemingly benign management decisions for parks can also act as barriers or disincentives to particular groups or individuals. Low et al (2009) found that fences erected for ecological reasons were perceived by the poorer, east-side users of Brooklyn's Prospect Park as a barrier to use, and Latino users, in particular, saw them as a sign of official neglect, equating them with danger, especially for women.

Fourth, engage in planning processes that invite more input from people and communities in which parks are to be built. How and where parks come to be should not be solely informed by those who own homes in nearby areas; it should also – and perhaps primarily – solicit participation from people who live near these, and not only homeowners but also renters and those who move around on transit and on foot.

Cities with available and accessible open space infrastructure prove more resilient because through it they promote greater health and opportunity for more of its residents. The current pandemic, like past pandemics, demonstrate that how we design, build, program, and grant access to our public space infrastructure is a matter of social justice, of life and death. When there is no Plan A in the form of a coordinated policy response, public space infrastructure is an essential Plan B.

PART II

Public Space and Human Well-Being

How Can Inequalities in Access to Green Space be Addressed in a Post-Pandemic World? Lessons from London

Meredith Whitten and Peter Massini

Introduction

Parks and green spaces have long featured prominently in city design and planning. Although once valued as a 'rejuvenative antidote to the city itself' (Pincetl and Gearin, 2005: 366), today green space is recognized as integral to the ecological, social, and economic functioning of cities. As global urbanization continues and cities grow more dense, congested, and polluted, providing healthy, liveable urban environments has become increasingly important. As such, delivering sufficient green space is a key objective for cities worldwide.

The value of green space has been underscored during the COVID-19 pandemic, as these spaces were some of the few places people could safely go to during lockdowns. Visiting green spaces became essential for getting daily exercise and combating social isolation. But, the pandemic also has highlighted the unequal provision of green space across builds a network of greener civic spaces that connect to and supplement existing parks.

Recent urban greening policies reflect an evolution of thinking about London's urban ecology that has moved from a focus on simply protecting existing green space to ensuring the benefits of green space are manifest within the built environment. These policy shifts were motivated primarily by managing the risks of climate change, which poses a significant threat to London's resilience. Recently, however, public health issues have become more significant drivers of urban greening policy and practice. COVID-19 has further thrown this into sharp focus.

Liveable Neighbourhoods

In 2018, London introduced the Liveable Neighbourhoods program to improve the local environment by transforming the city's streets into places of active travel. As part of a broader Healthy Streets approach set out in the Mayor's Transport Strategy to change how people move about the city, Liveable Neighbourhoods invests in long-term local schemes that reduce car trips and provide more sustainable travel options, including walking, cycling, and public transport (GLA, 2018b).

Projects, which are expected to include a mode shift away from private vehicles, involve creating green spaces, adding cycling infrastructure, redesigning junctions, and widening walking routes. The program's broad design allows for flexibility to accommodate a wide range of projects across London neighborhoods, which have distinct characteristics and challenges (Transport for London (TfL), 2019).

As an immediate response to the impact of COVID-19, the need to encourage social distancing on London's high streets led to the initiation of the Streetspace for London Plan, which has implemented hundreds of temporary measures to reduce traffic and promote walking and cycling. These are precursors to more permanent solutions implemented through acceleration of the

Liveable Neighbourhoods approach as London transitions to the new normal of the post-COVID-19 city.

Yet, Liveable Neighbourhood projects have not been problem-free. Several boroughs have reversed or paused their initiatives after some residents and businesses expressed opposition. Arguments against the schemes contend they can exacerbate inequalities, with those living in more affluent central neighborhoods with better public transport provision benefiting at the expense of residents in the poorer suburbs who are dependent on their cars or unable to walk or cycle to workplaces, schools, and other destinations.

Urban greening

The new London Plan has introduced the Urban Greening Factor (UGF) as part of a new Urban Greening policy. As a planning tool, the UGF provides a means for ensuring new developments contain an appropriate amount of on-site greening by setting targets for how green a project should be. Each landscape element – such as a tree, green roof, or rain garden – is assigned a factor between zero and one; natural elements score higher, while sealed surfaces score zero (GLA, 2021). The UGF enables local authorities to encourage particular green infrastructure interventions. For example, those concerned about flooding can confer a higher factor for sustainable drainage elements (see Figure 9.1). The policy encourages developers to integrate greening into projects at the start of the design process and provides flexibility to adapt their designs if circumstances change (Massini and Smith, 2018).

The UGF aims to enhance the functionality of urban greening by shifting the use of green elements from a passive adornment in development schemes to essential working landscapes. This is particularly impactful as an area grows denser, as embedding green infrastructure into development can offset some adverse impacts resulting from increased pressure on land use (Massini and Smith, 2018). More localized UGF policies could target

Figure 9.1: Kidbrooke Village sustainable urban drainage system (SUDS), Royal Borough of Greenwich, London

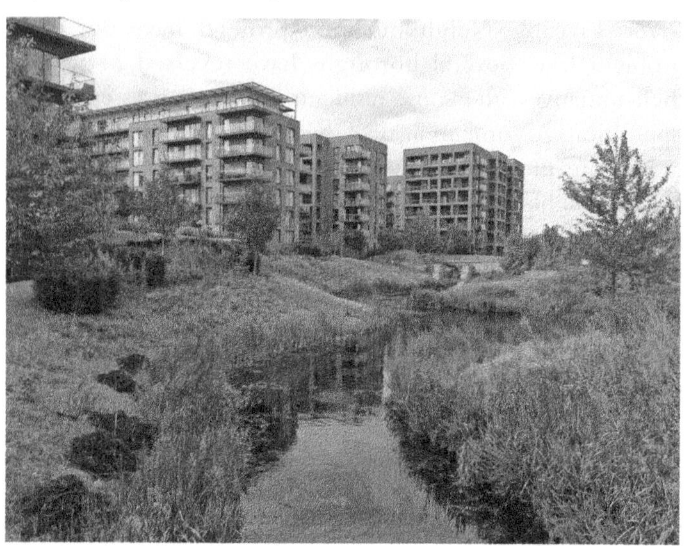

Source: Peter Massini

neighborhoods that are most deficient in access to green space, thus helping to address existing health inequalities.

This approach requires a shift from longstanding conceptualizations of green space as merely public parks to recognition of the potential benefits that a more diverse range of green elements can deliver in increasingly dense urban areas. It can increase the greening of those areas where creating new parks is unachievable. However, it is reliant on a trade-off between creating features that improve flood prevention, air and water filtration, urban cooling, and biodiversity – which all contribute to positive health outcomes – and more conventional green space interventions that can accommodate activities, such as team sports and dog walking. Enhancing urban greening through urban regeneration can also shift more of the provision of urban greening to the private sector, which further raises issues of access and inequalities and the risk of gentrification.

Discussion

Although London has provided strong protection for its expansive green space network, a growing population and land-use policies favoring high-density development curtail opportunities to deliver new conventional green spaces (Whitten, 2020). At the same time, the increasingly urgent threats of climate change, public health, and loss of biodiversity have deepened pressure to leverage the comprehensive benefits urban green space provides. Further, COVID-19 has intensified demand to prioritize tackling longstanding inequalities in access to green spaces and the positive health outcomes they provide.

Pre-pandemic, London had already begun implementing a new approach to greening the urban environment. Supplementing the traditional approach of conventional features, such as parks, for delivering green space, London has adopted an ambitious urban greening policy and proactive initiatives, including the UGF and Liveable Neighbourhoods. This approach represents a more efficient use of the policy and funding levers available to deliver enhanced urban greening more quickly.

Yet, these approaches should not be implemented as a matter of parks versus urban greening. Although these initiatives help mitigate some of the disadvantages of insufficient access to green space, they do not eliminate them. Protecting the existing network of public parks is a prerequisite, and a network of green space of multiple shapes, sizes, and uses is needed to address health and environmental inequities. The urban greening approach simply reflects the realities of providing green space in urban areas already, and increasingly, spatially constrained by density.

Rather than reacting to issues raised by the pandemic by introducing rushed and impractical schemes, London is able

London Legacy Development Corporation (2020) *Lockdown Love Makes the Park Grow Stronger, Study Shows.* www.queenelizabetholympicpark.co.uk/news/news-articles/2020/06/lockdown-love-makes-the-park-grow-stronger-study-shows

Massini, P. and Smith, H. (2018) *PERFECT Expert Paper 2: Planning for Green Infrastructure – the Green Space Factor and Learning from Europe.* www.interregeurope.eu/fileadmin/user_upload/tx_tevprojects/library/file_1551105810.pdf

Natural England (2020) *Monitor of Engagement with the Natural Environment (MENE).* www.gov.uk/government/collections/monitor-of-engagement-with-the-natural-environment-survey-purpose-and-results

The Nursery Research and Planning Ltd (2020) *London Legacy Development Corporation: Queen Elizabeth Olympic Park – Covid Research.* www.parksleisure.com.au/includes/download.ashx?ID=157791

Office for National Statistics (2020) *Access to Garden Spaces: England.* www.ons.gov.uk/economy/environmentalaccounts/methodologies/accesstogardenspacesengland

Pincetl, S. and Gearin, E. (2005) 'The reinvention of public green space'. *Urban Geography*, 26(5): 365–84.

Public Health England (2020) *Improving Access to Greenspace: A New Review for 2020.* https://assets.publishing.service.gov.uk/government/uploads/system/uploads/attachment_data/file/904439/Improving_access_to_greenspace_2020_review.pdf

Transport for London (2019) *Liveable Neighbourhoods Programme Guidance.* http://content.tfl.gov.uk/tfl-liveable-neighbourhood-guidance.pdf

Whitten, M. (2020) 'Contesting longstanding conceptualisations of urban green space', in N. Dempsey and J. Dobson (eds) *Naturally Challenged: Contested Perceptions and Practices in Urban Green Spaces.* Cham, Switzerland: Springer, pp 87–116.

TEN

America Under COVID-19: The Plight of the Old

Setha Low and Anastasia Loukaitou-Sideris

Introduction

Older adults represent the fastest-growing population segment in the US and many other cities of the Global North (United Nations, 2019), thanks to longer life spans and advancements in medicine. But along with the longer life expectancy come also challenges. Deteriorating physical health, death of a spouse or partner, and living alone make older adults particularly vulnerable to social isolation and loneliness (Victor and Bowling, 2012; see also Volume 4, Chapter Ten). Indeed, the likelihood of living alone increases with age, and this is particularly true for women (Nies and McEwen, 2015). Social isolation often leads to deteriorating mental and physical health (Luanaigh and Lawlor, 2008), including depression, decreases in cognitive functioning, cardiovascular disease, and even mortality (Courtin and Knapp, 2015).

One aspect of counteracting and lessening social isolation is to have opportunities and neighborhood places to go to, to meet, and communicate with others (see also Chapter Eleven, this volume). Being able to walk to the neighborhood grocery store or park not only helps older adults accomplish activities of daily living (ADLs) but also facilitates their social well-being and social needs (Clarke and Gallagher, 2013). Therefore, the built environment – and in particular its public places and 'third spaces' – interacts with the social environment (Kweon et al, 1998) and influences older adults' health and well-being (World Health Organization, 2015).

But the COVID-19 pandemic has been brutal for older adults. Not only has it decimated their lives, but it has also increased the fear among the living of accessing public spaces, thus furthering their social isolation. As researchers of public space and aging from New York City and Los Angeles, we have talked with a number of older adults in our cities, who have been spared from the pandemic but remain stuck at home. One of them, Rebecca, 65, lives in a low-rise building in Brooklyn. She avoids the elevator in case other people use it and takes the stairs; but when she arrives at the street, it is too crowded to safely walk to the nearby park. One early morning she ventured out to Prospect Park, but found it crowded with young people not wearing masks and just turned around and went home. Eighty-year-old Harold, who lives near Times Square, where automobile traffic has been rerouted, cannot find a place to rest because chairs have been removed to discourage gathering. He lives too far to walk to a park and worries about taking the subway to visit one. A Latina house cleaner, Maria, 70, hopes to restart her job in Los Angeles, but worries about riding the bus that would bring her to the Larchmond neighborhood, where she works.

We are concerned that not much thought has gone into how these and many other vulnerable older adults can again use some critical settings of their everyday life: their neighborhood's public spaces. People over 65 are considered 'senior citizens' in the US but represent an afterthought on the part of policy makers, who by their actions or inertia are contributing to high levels of mortality and feelings of desperation and social isolation among seniors. The consequences of oversight, the fear of death, increased stigma and discrimination, and the impacts of physical distancing and social isolation are adding to their anxiety, loneliness, and well-being.

The plight of the old is exacerbated by increasing inequities in terms of health and economic security, at the same time that the numbers of people over 65 are expanding in the US and globally. And of course, certain subgroups of older adults witness greater disparities. Sixteen percent of women and 12 percent of men 65 or older in the US live at or below the poverty level. Older people of color experience poverty at significantly higher rates than their White counterparts (US Census Bureau, 2019). And it is exactly from these individuals – poor, minority, and old – that the COVID-19 pandemic is taking its highest toll (Centers for Disease Control and Prevention (CDC), 2020).

We believe that there needs to be a special recognition of the rights of older people and thoughtful actions to mediate the psychological and social impacts of the pandemic. In this chapter, we first lay out the scope of the problem and the multiple injustices towards older people in US cities, which have been accentuated by the pandemic. We then turn to discuss some suggestions for a better future of our cities and public spaces that takes into account the well-being of older adults (see also Volume 1, Chapter Nineteen).

The scope of the problem

Natural diseases typically affect the old in disproportionately higher amounts than the younger population, because of their greater physical, economic, and social vulnerabilities. The deadly heatwave that hit Chicago in the summer of 1995 killed hundreds of older people who were socially isolated at their homes (Klinenberg, 2015). Similarly, nearly 40 percent of the victims of Hurricane Katrina were over 71 (National Public Radio (NPR), 2006); because of limited mobility many of them were trapped in their homes, when the city flooded. The impact of COVID-19 on the older population is not different.

time in their neighborhood parks, or sit and read a book on a park bench. While the beaches, hiking trails, and other nature spaces at the edges of the city have re-opened, these are not the spaces that older adults can easily reach or use. Other 'third places' where elders could previously socialize – barbershops, community gardens, mall food courts, old-fashioned cafeterias – are also slowly re-opening, but many older adults are still scared to use them. The fear of infection looms so large that their participation in daily activities will be slow or non-existent without interventions in public space policies and practices.

Lack of virtual public space: no Zoom meetings for the old. The digital divide has become even bigger under COVID-19. Connecting virtually with friends and family or shopping online is not an option for many older people living alone, who do not have Wi-Fi services or simply do not know how to use them. The assumption that everyone has access to virtual communication systems ignores the levels of poverty and deprivation found among older people who live on limited social security and fixed incomes. The technology and internet speeds necessary to enable Zoom or webinar communication is expensive and difficult to use for many older people.

How can we then alleviate the plight of older people in the post-pandemic era? How can we reopen cities with the needs and fears of older adults in mind?

The response: rethinking cities with older adults in mind

As we are getting ready to reclaim public spaces in our cities, we also have to adapt to the new normal of physical distancing. Some spatial interventions will be helpful. For example, many stores have created special hours for older patrons to shop without the fear of bumping into crowds. But they also need to retrofit their parking lots and waiting areas with more seating and shade, that would allow older people to wait in line comfortably, if they have to.

Privileging the old and most vulnerable citizens in parks and on public transit can also be accomplished by designating benches and special compartments on transit vehicles for their exclusive use. Why not designate 'seniors only' settings at popular parks and beaches for the exclusive use of older adults, with benches spaced safely apart for socializing? Or allot the first car of every subway train and the front section near the driver in every bus for vulnerable populations.

The street system may be more difficult to rearrange in ways that offer safe walking and shopping for seniors. In New York City, however, Mayor de Blasio has already dedicated seven miles of streets to pedestrians and cyclists and plans to open up 100 miles in all to promote physical distancing during the pandemic. A similar strategy can also work in Los Angeles, a city that has a plethora of streets for cars, but narrow and often non-existent sidewalks for pedestrians. Open streets add public spaces for walking in cities and counteract sidewalk crowding, but to encourage walking among older adults, they also need to be retrofitted with benches for resting and comfort, and trees for shade.

We are not alone in our thinking. There have been numerous outcries against the closing of parks and arguments about public green spaces being good both for the mind and for the body (Tufekci, 2020). But there has been no comprehensive framework or guidance for allocating public space for those who need it the most. Planners and public space managers might consider a new set of public space principles as they look to the future where contagion and vulnerability to disease is paramount.

Four principles for the allocation of public space for the vulnerable

We propose four principles to allocate public space that considers the needs of vulnerable groups during this historical moment. The first principle asks that we reconsider the distribution of space for activities and people. A fair distribution of space is the hallmark of just public space planning and is usually thought about in terms of meeting the needs of all people, fairly and equally (Low and Iveson, 2016). An equitable distribution of public open space is foundational to democratic and health practices. However, spatial distribution needs to be reconsidered under a pandemic to prioritize the needs of older and more vulnerable groups, who may not be able to use collective space but might benefit from specific designations of places designed and protected for their needs. One question that lingers, however, when considering spatial interventions is whether spatial protections will exacerbate social segregation and inequalities in unintended ways. We believe that the answer is to provide options to older people that are not mutually exclusive, offering the choice of using these protections or not, as they see fit.

The second principle in the allocation of public space relates to temporality. It considers a public space as a location that can be used differently over time. All public spaces have a temporal rhythm with different people and activities transforming them throughout the day and night. In fact, the most successful Latin American plazas provide a 'work space' for retired men reading their newspaper in early morning; a 'play space' for school children who arrive later, a 'social space' for mothers who come to rest after shopping, later in the day, and a 'hip space or courting space' for youth arriving to meet friends, play soccer, or dance in the evening (Low, 2017). We can consider using the temporal dimension of public space as a way to allocate specific times in early morning, when some parks would open earlier for 'older adults only', thus creating spaces they can venture to, without the fear of crowds and families.

Our third principle relates to the use of digital and smart technologies in public space. Such technologies have become popular in recent years helping to monitor humidity, water usage, and environmental damage in parks; offering free Wi-Fi or providing a surveillance apparatus to ensure physical safety

(Loukaitou-Sideris et al, 2018). While increased surveillance and policing in public space are problematic, and can also be discriminatory, it is important to consider what other smart technologies can provide to vulnerable populations. For one, mobile communication devices are helpful to older adults reaching out for help while in public space; solar shade umbrellas tracking the sun can offer better shade protection in very hot weather; while smart street/park benches can provide heated, frost-free, and comfortable seating surfaces in cold weather. Waiting for buses or standing in line on hot sidewalks without adequate shade poses risks especially to seniors, thus new tensile technologies with solar-reflecting materials and cool pavements could be used for better comfort in public spaces.

The fourth principle relates to the provision of a psychologically positive and inclusive atmosphere, where older adults can feel safe and welcome. The stigma of being old and vulnerable has always been a deterrent to the use of public space. With COVID-19, it has become even more important to signal that public spaces are designed to safely accommodate seniors' needs and sensitivities. We have written elsewhere that a welcoming public space for older adults needs to be physically and psychologically accessible, offering age-friendly design and programming, opportunities for low-impact physical activities, as well as settings for social interaction (Loukaitou-Sideris, 2020). Much has also been written about the design of public space for people of different abilities and these ideas offer ways to intervene that not only help draw older adults into public spaces, but also generate design changes that improve the physical and social environment and make it more inclusive for everyone.

These four principles are only a first step towards imagining a better future, even in a world where contagion and disease become frequent risks. As we are taking stock and assessing the effectiveness of our efforts against the pandemic, and looking to a period of reorganizing our built environment and social world, we should also reconsider how we treat the

Whalen, A. (2020) 'What is "Boomer Remover" and why is it making people so angry?' *Newsweek*, March 13. Retrieved from: www.newsweek.com/boomer-remover-meme-trends-virus-coronavirus-social-media-COVID-19-baby-boomers-1492190

World Health Organization (2015) *World Report on Aging and Health.* Geneva: WHO Press.

ELEVEN

Exploring Older Adults' Experiences of Urban Space in the COVID-19 Lockdowns: Dutch and British Perspectives

Tess Osborne, Arlinde Dul, and Louise Meijering

Introduction

During the COVID-19 pandemic and the consequential lockdowns, the importance of urban neighborhoods as public spaces for people in general, and older adults in particular, has increased (see also Chapter Ten, this volume). This importance has increased because the lockdowns forced/encouraged people to spend the majority of their time at home, only leaving to get some fresh air or go shopping, both activities that often take place locally. In this chapter, we explore various areas in urban neighborhoods in which older adults engage most, and how experiences of service use and green and blue space have been impacted.

For older adults, the local neighborhood typically is an important place. It is where they undertake the majority of their daily activities (such as socializing, shopping, and exercising) and thus experience a strong sense of belonging and attachment (Smith, 2009; Buffel et al, 2014). This sense of belonging is a fundamental element of 'ageing in place' which, in turn, is important to well-being in later life (Wiles et al, 2012): when older adults live in a neighborhood, they typically have a relatively strong local social network, and know how, when, and with whom to engage with its spaces (Boyle et al, 2015).

Another key element for older adults in urban neighborhoods is the quantity and quality of amenities available, such as supermarkets, green space, and health care facilities. Aside from the functional needs of the amenities, spaces such as gardens, parks, ponds, and waterfronts are considered to have restorative and even 'therapeutic' qualities (Korpela et al, 2010; Bell et al, 2017): people go there to relax, to spend time on their own (or with other people) away from the hustle and bustle of urban life. More specifically, green and blue space have been found to positively affect perceived mental, physical, and social health in later life, but complicating these positive effects are negative experiences around safety and accessibility (Finlay et al, 2015). To ensure positive ageing in place, these amenities need to be freely accessible and safe for older adults (Van Hoven and Meijering, 2019). However, even if services are nearby, they may not always be accessible for those who use mobility aids or may not be deemed safe (Van Hoven and Meijering, 2019).

Methodology and contexts

This study is part of Meaningful Mobility (2019–24) project which explores mobility patterns and experiences in later life. From the project, 38 older adults (21 Lancashire, UK, and 17 Northern Netherlands), ranging in age from 59 to 82, were recruited for an interview about their everyday experiences and quality of life during the lockdowns. Although the age categorization of 'vulnerable', in relation to COVID-19, differed between the UK and the Netherlands (60+ and 70+ respectively), it is important to note that not all of the participants in this study considered themselves 'vulnerable', but nevertheless chose to or were forced to change their behavior. As such, the participants had different characteristics in terms of health status, living arrangements, location, and lifestyle. Interviews were held via telephone in the native language of the participants and lasted approximately 30 to 60 minutes.

Lancashire and the Northern Netherlands had lower infection numbers compared to other regions in the country meaning that the areas are not the focus of the outbreak, but still bound to the lockdown measures detailed by the governments (National Institute for Public Health and the Environment (RIVM), 2020; Office for National Statistics (ONS), 2020). The Netherlands implemented an 'intelligent lockdown', which included the closure of schools, restaurants and bars, services involving direct contact (for example hairdressers), and public places (for example libraries and museums). A 1.5m person-to-person distancing was encouraged, and while outside activities were permitted it could only be with three or fewer persons, and people were advised to work from home. Compared to the Dutch measures, the UK implemented an obligated person-to-person distance of 2m and people's outside mobility was limited to an hour of exercise or daily essential needs, such as grocery shopping. In both countries, all services were closed except for essential amenities including food retailers and pharmacies among others.

Everyday experiences of lockdown in the UK and the Netherlands

The lockdown measures in both countries had significant implications on the older adults' experiences of their local community and neighborhood since their mobility was restricted to their immediate environments, such as their home and their road/apartment block (see also Volume 1, Chapter Nineteen).

as nature reserves and the surrounding countryside: "There's a lot, there's lots of lovely landscape 'round us. So, I go out every other day, or so and I'll spend two [or] three hours. So, it's very pleasant in the sunshine" (Mr Chapman, UK). Yet the increased popularity of natural spaces in the UK and the Netherlands during lockdown meant that these green spaces had increasing numbers of visitors, and were seen by the older adults to be unsafe and therefore avoided:

> 'I live a hundred meters from the forest and that is why I can always go for a walk here in the area. And I just notice […] that it is getting busier and busier. In the beginning when I walked there I saw very few people and now you see more and more. I have to be careful.'
> (Mr Kuipers, NL)

So, while the participants enjoyed the green spaces in their neighborhoods, the increased popularity of these spaces meant that they avoided these spaces or engaged with them cautiously or at times when they knew it would be quiet. Thus, the older adults could not fully engage with all the public space in their local neighborhoods, like they did prior to the pandemic.

Conclusion

In this chapter, we explored the similarities and differences in the lockdown experiences of older adults in urban neighborhoods in the UK and the Netherlands. In both countries, we found that everyday experiences became more localized, and that participants concentrated their (food) shopping on one day a week. A notable difference between the two countries was that participants in the UK in particular avoided the city center, as they thought it would be crowded, which Dutch participants did not. However, those UK participants who went into town, described it as a ghost town and rather eerie. In the Netherlands, participants similarly described inner city experiences as surreal because the streets were deserted. The green spaces in and around the city, however, were much busier than the city center. It is already well established that green space was extremely important during the lockdowns (Slater et al, 2020), yet we have shown that the increased popularity for green space can be an impediment for older adults. With an increased number of people in and using green space, the participants reported that they felt unsafe using these spaces because of the crowding, and therefore began to avoid them. Our data has shown that the shift in scale and avoidance strategies has changed the ways older adults engage with public space. The main drive behind these changes is the perceptions of safety for themselves and others, such as vulnerable members in their household, or those they care for.

The COVID-19 lockdown measures have had major impacts on everyday life, especially for older adults. We have shown that local urban neighborhoods have become even more important spaces for older adults both in the UK and the Netherlands. The participants, as a result of the perceived risk of crowds and busy spaces, often chose to be in and interact with spaces a short distance from their homes, such as local shops, green space, and their neighborhood. While this may imply that older adults were reduced in their mobility, we have shown that for many it has also been a positive experience since it has enriched their social interactions around the immediate neighborhood, and led them to discover new local shops. Therefore, the pandemic may have a positive impact upon ageing in place in the long run, since it has enabled older adults to renew and foster their connections and social worlds in their local areas (see also Volume 2, Chapter Eleven).

Funding statement

The authors would like to acknowledge the funding they have received from the European Research Council (ERC) under the European Union's Horizon 2020 research and innovation program (*Meaningful Mobility*, Grant Agreement No. 802202).

References

Bell, S.L., Wheeler, B.W. and Phoenix, C. (2017) 'Using geo-narratives to explore the diverse temporalities of therapeutic landscapes: perspectives from "green" and "blue" settings'. *Annals of the Association of American Geographers*, 107(1): 93–108.

Boyle, A., Wiles, J.L. and Kearns, R. (2015) 'Rethinking ageing in place: the "people" and "place" nexus'. *Progress in Human Geography*, 34(12): 1495–511.

Buffel, T., de Donder, L., Phillipson, C., de Witte, N., Dury, S. and Verté, D. (2014) 'Place attachment among older adults living in four communities in Flanders, Belgium'. *Housing Studies*, 29(6): 800–22.

Finlay, L., Franke, T., McKay, H. and Sims-Gould, J. (2015) 'Therapeutic landscapes and wellbeing in later life: impacts of blue and green spaces for older adults'. *Health & Place*, 34: 97–106.

Korpela, K.M., Ylén, M., Tyrväinen, L. and Silvennoinen, H. (2010) 'Favorite green, waterside and urban environments, restorative experiences and perceived health in Finland'. *Health Promotion International*, 25(2): 200–09.

National Institute for Public Health and the Environment (RIVM) (2020) *Current information about COVID-19.* Retrieved from: www.rivm.nl/en/novel-coronavirus-covid-19/current-information

Office for National Statistics (ONS) (2020) *Coronavirus (COVID-19) in the UK.* Retrieved from: https://coronavirus.data.gov.uk/#category=regions&map=rate

Slater, S.J., Chrisiana, R.W. and Gustat, J. (2020) 'Recommendations for keeping parks and green space accessible for mental and physical health during COVID-19 and other pandemics'. *Preventing Chronic Disease*, 17, http://dx.doi.org/10.5888/pcd17.200204

Smith, A.E. (2009) *Ageing in Urban Neighbourhoods. Place Attachment and Social Exclusion.* Bristol: Policy Press.

Van Hoven, B. and Meijering, L. (2019) 'Mundane mobilities in later life: exploring experiences of everyday trip-making by older adults in a Dutch urban neighbourhood'. *Research in Transportation Business & Management*, 30: 100375.

Wiles, J.L., Leibing, A., Guberman, N., Reeve, J. and Allen, R.E.S. (2012) 'The meaning of "ageing in place" to older people'. *The Gerontologist*, 52(3): 357–66.

a national public infrastructure crippled by ten years of austerity and hollowing out of library services (Corble, 2019).

This chapter starts with an overview of the national pictures of British and Dutch public libraries before and during the COVID-19 pandemic, after which we discuss two important changes in: 1) the library's functioning and 2) the nature of librarianship. It is based on interviews with seven anonymized staff members (three in NL, four in UK) and UK public library worker and campaigner Alan Wylie, who sits on the national 'Cultural Renewal Taskforce' for steering library services through the COVID-19 crisis. These interviews took place within the framework of our volunteering-as-research practices that already started in the years prior to the pandemic, respectively in a single library in a suburban context of Utrecht (NL) and a library service including multiple sites in a London borough (UK). Through this data we address the question of what the public library is for, when services are stripped back to the bare functional minimum of information provision, and their vital social spaces and infrastructures are suspended as the impact of both neoliberalism and the pandemic takes its toll on public life.

Crisis-upon-crisis

It is well-evidenced that libraries are essential lifelines for low-income, isolated, or marginalized people (Jaeger et al, 2014), and during a global pandemic such lifelines are more critical than ever.[1] Public libraries facilitate digital access and support for citizens to access essential online welfare services and are often the only source of both face-to-face and online connection for a significant portion of the population,[2] as well as providing the core offer of supporting literacy and cultural development. However, as with many (public) institutions, public libraries are heavily impacted by the COVID-19 crisis, though the hardest hit might be yet to come as most subsidies for 2020 were already granted before the pandemic started.

Dutch libraries rely for a large part (82 percent in 2018) on (mostly municipal) subsidies, amounting to 407 million in 2018.[3] As government budgets are expected to be strained in response to the COVID-19 crisis, the library's income is likely to reduce significantly in the future. However, it is important to note that this sense of decline already pre-existed COVID-19. Between 2014 and 2018, there has been a decrease in subsidies (-5 percent), the number of library locations (-27 percent) and adult membership (-12 percent) in the Netherlands.[4]

In the UK public libraries are also reliant on public subsidy, and central government puts legal obligations on local governments to provide 'a comprehensive and efficient library services to all persons desiring to make use thereof' (Public Libraries and Museums Act 1964).[5] The last decade of austerity has thrown the UK public library network into crisis, as successive rounds of funding cuts have hollowed out services. Despite widespread local and national campaigns to save libraries from cuts and closures, since 2009–10 local authority spending on neighborhood services was reduced by 28 percent, with public libraries taking the biggest financial hit with a cut of 41 percent, and these cuts have been larger in more deprived areas of the UK.[6] In the same period, 17 percent of libraries have closed and the number of professional employees in UK public libraries fell by 38 percent, while the number of (largely untrained) volunteers delivering library services rose by 187 percent.[7]

This crisis situation is also felt in our two investigated cases. Our Dutch case is the only library left in town; two other locations were closed due to budget cuts. It is staffed by two part-time librarians assisted by a pool of 15 volunteers. When faced with further cuts, the library's director responded to the alderman: 'Why don't you close this library too and free me from the responsibility to run it with too limited means? We already work on a "minimum scenario", further budget cuts are impossible.' Fortunately, the municipal subsidy was not strained since. However, future prospects look bleak, as the municipality announced that COVID-19 forces them to make cutbacks, and the library was already framed as 'extra' the town could do without.

Our UK case is a public library service in an inner borough of London with significant socio-economic deprivation and a young and ethnically diverse population. The service has been profoundly affected by a decade of austerity: in 2010 it had one central library and 12 branch libraries – today it has only three professionally staffed 'hub' libraries, one largely self-service council-run library, and nine community-managed branch libraries which receive no statutory funding and are staffed by volunteers, but remain stocked by council-owned circulating book stock through a networked community liaison model.

Therefore, there already was a 'hollowing out' and 'deprofessionalization' of library spaces and services (Robertson and McMenemy, 2020) in both countries prior to the pandemic. As one UK library manager argues, 'We fight every day to keep the service alive. It feels like a war zone. Library leaders have battle scars on their backs.'[8] At the same time, adult illiteracy is alarmingly high; 18 percent in the Netherlands[9] and 16 percent in the UK.[10] We can thus speak of a crisis-upon-crisis situation, which perpetuates social injustice for the most vulnerable of library users and workers, whose lives and livelihoods depend on social investment in libraries as spaces of care. Despite this injustice, there is a policy narrative in the UK that posits COVID-19 as an 'opportunity' for libraries to play an essential part in local recovery and continue to reinvent themselves as hubs for partnership and collaboration using neoliberal business models and voluntary labor.[11]

Changing function of the library

It is increasingly acknowledged that public libraries are more than 'Habermasian' information infrastructures facilitating literacy, but also vital social infrastructures (Klinenberg, 2018). According to the Dutch library law of 2015, providing knowledge and information is only one of the five functions libraries should fulfill, alongside, for example, organizing encounter and debate. UK legislation is less explicit on the socio-cultural functions of public libraries, however, the national charity that supports strategic library service development defines the four 'Universal Library Offers' as 1) reading, 2) digital and information, 3) culture and creativity, and 4) health and well-being.[12]

In 2017–18, the majority of people using UK public library services were Black, Asian or Minority Ethnic and unemployed, and 34 percent of users were adults with long-term illness or disability.[13] UK libraries are also a key service that can bridge the nation's significant digital divide, since 10 percent of the adult population have either never or rarely used the internet and 16 percent are unable to use the internet without assistance and rely on public library services to gain online access and support.[14] As sites of such vital social and digital inclusion, it is perhaps not surprising that libraries were one of the last public infrastructures to close their doors in the UK's response to COVID-19, much to the concern of many vulnerable library workers.[15]

At the first height of the pandemic, library buildings in both countries were fully closed for at least two months, during which a plethora of online activities emerged such as virtual reading group and storytime sessions, increasing online collection access, and a range of outreach activities for vulnerable citizens.[16] During the lockdown, digital membership of UK libraries grew by 600 percent and e-book lending statistics quadrupled.[17] Not all UK public library staff were able to focus on such digital services during lockdown, however, since many were redeployed into local authority COVID-19 response teams, delivering services such as crisis helplines, social care outreach, and in some cases even working in cemeteries to help manage the mounting death toll (Interview Alan, 2020). Once some of the lockdown measures were eased, many UK and Dutch libraries offered a 'click-and-collect' option,

the limits of public librarianship, these workers focused on developing a program of online literacy and storytelling videos.

After being allowed to reopen, the professional duties of library workers changed again. Instead of acting as social infrastructures, staff were now occupied by enacting very strict protocols, such as organizing the three-day book quarantine and sterilizing shopping baskets. In mid-June, after the initial happiness of being allowed to reopen had faded away, Linda complained that she "might as well work in Albert Heijn [a Dutch supermarket]", as she would be cleaning baskets there also. She immediately added that disinfecting the library is an important task she gladly performs, but that everything that gave her job challenge and content is now gone – with little prospects that organizing social activities is allowed anytime soon. Consequently, it is very likely that some of the organized activities, like the lunch meetings for lonely elderly, will be difficult to rebuild after social restrictions are eased. Norcup (2017) shows the difficulties of maintaining such architectures of sociability in the long run under 'normal' circumstances, let alone in times of a pandemic.

Conclusion: Loss-upon-loss

COVID-19 has worsened an already precarious situation for public libraries, adding loss-upon-loss for the vital roles they fulfill as a social contract. As Robinson and Sheldon (2019) argue, bearing witness to such loss is important for our understanding of the everyday ways in which libraries matter. The current crisis could be the final nail in the coffin of some public libraries. Indeed our UK case fears for its future to operate at all, since it has lost the small income it had from renting out the space to community groups and selling second-hand books, and the expensive utility bills are mounting up without means to pay.

Daunting though this situation certainly is, it also shows us we desperately need robust public institutions, and not only in the domain of public health. If anything, our findings show that libraries have not become obsolete, even if their physical functioning is limited to click-and-collect. Though librarians' tasks have changed from organizing lunch meetings and helping with homework to sterilizing baskets, offering online assistance, and sometimes even being re-deployed to other council work, spaces and relations of care still exist in and through the library and its staff.

Yet, the dominant narrative, at least in the UK, of seeing the COVID-19 crisis as an 'opportunity' for libraries to show their value as essential lifelines is problematic. As Alan puts it:

'It's as if the last ten years of austerity hasn't happened. All this rhetoric of COVID[-19] being an opportunity for libraries to reinvent themselves – I get the feeling that it's just another round of moving libraries towards a neoliberal hub model ... there's no "new normal" as they say – the only thing that's "normal" is gearing up for the next round of cuts.'

When asked where the hope lies for the future, Alan replied that what keeps him going is continuing to provide for the library community and fight for the rights of his fellow library workers. The other library staff we spoke to confirmed a sense of how struggling through the working conditions of the pandemic together created a renewed sense of what a public library is for: a space of care, no matter how fragile, hidden or restricted the infrastructures may now be.

Notes

[1]   www.bbc.co.uk/news/uk-england-suffolk-53312324

[2]   In 2018, 10 percent of the UK's adult population were internet non-users, which raises grave concerns for these citizens' access to public health information and welfare services without access to public libraries (Watts, 2020).

[3]   www.rijksoverheid.nl/documenten/rapporten/2020/02/11/bijlage-2-kwink-eindrapport-evaluatie-wsob

4   www.rijksoverheid.nl/documenten/rapporten/2020/02/11/bijlage-2-kwink-eindrapport-evaluatie-wsob

5   www.legislation.gov.uk/ukpga/1964/75

6   www.instituteforgovernment.org.uk/publication/performance-tracker-2019/neighbourhood-services

7   www.instituteforgovernment.org.uk/publication/performance-tracker-2019/neighbourhood-services

8   www.thebookseller.com/news/public-library-sector-war-zone-678926

9   www.lezenenschrijven.nl/over-laaggeletterdheid/feiten-cijfers? gcl id=EAIaIQobChMIo7DQ6aqY6wIVBbd3Ch10ag4-EAAYAi AAEgIZyvD_BwE

10 https://literacytrust.org.uk/parents-and-families/adult-literacy/

11 https://communitylibrariesnetwork.wordpress.com/2020/09/25/libraries-as-the-hub-of-the-21st-century-community/

12 www.librariesconnected.org.uk/page/universal-library-offers

13 www.gov.uk/government/statistics/taking-part-201819-statistical-release

14 www.librariesconnected.org.uk/page/universal-library-offers

15 https://dontprivatiselibraries.blogspot.com/2020/04/close-libraries.html

16 www.bibliotheekinzicht.nl/dossiers/de-bibliotheek-in-coronatijd

17 www.librariesconnected.org.uk/resource/libraries-essential-part-local-recovery

References

Aptekar, S. (2019) 'The public library as resistive space in the neo-liberal city'. *City & Community*, 18(4): 1203–19.

Barniskis, S.C. (2016) 'Access and express: professional perspectives on public library makerspaces and intellectual freedom'. *Public Library Quarterly*, 35(2): 103–25.

Corble, A.R. (2019) *The Death and Life of English Public Libraries: Infrastructural Practices and Value in a Time of Crisis.* Doctoral thesis, Goldsmiths, University of London. http://research.gold.ac.uk/26145/

Jaeger, P.T., Gorham, U., Bertot, J.C. and Sarin, L.C. (2014) *Public Libraries, Public Policies, and Political Processes: Serving and Transforming Communities in Times of Economic and Political Constraint.* Lanham: Rowman & Littlefield.

Klinenberg, E. (2018) *Palaces for the People: How to Build a More Equal and United Society.* London: The Bodley Head.

Mehta, A. (2010) *Overdue, Returned, and Missing: The Changing Stories of Boston's Chinatown Branch Library*. Doctoral thesis, Massachusetts Institute of Technology.

Norcup, J. (2017) '"Educate a woman and you educate a generation": performing geographies of learning, the public library and a pre-school parents' book club'. *Performance Research*, 22(1): 67–74.

Robertson, C. and McMenemy, D. (2020) 'The hollowing out of children's public library services in England from 2010 to 2016'. *Journal of Librarianship and Information Science*, 52(1): 91–105.

Robinson, K. (2014) *An Everyday Public? Placing Public Libraries in London and Berlin*. Doctoral thesis, The London School of Economics and Political Science (LSE). http://etheses.lse.ac.uk/3090/

Robinson, K. and Sheldon, R. (2019) 'Witnessing loss in the everyday: community buildings in austerity Britain'. *The Sociological Review*, 67(1): 111–25.

van Melik, R. (2020) 'Van boekenbieb naar volkspaleis'. *Geografie*, 29(3): 22–4.

Watts, G. (2020) 'COVID-19 and the digital divide in the UK'. *The Lancet Digital Health*, 2(8): e395–6. https://doi.org/10.1016/S2589-7500(20)30169-2

live in. Many residents' 'right to the city' (Lefebvre, 1968) is jeopardized and children are a group specially affected, mostly because their mobility and free use of public spaces encounter progressive restrictions.

Urban childhood is marked by a decrease in children's independent mobility and use of public spaces (Fyhri et al, 2011; Shaw et al, 2015). Children's daily lives tend to revolve around three indoor settings: home, school, and recreational institutions (Rasmussen, 2004; Sarmento, 2018). Hence, 'the playful dimension of the city' (Farné, 2017: 165) is being lost, and we know that children's play is an essential activity for their physical, social, and emotional development and well-being (Sarmento, 2018; Russel and Stenning, 2020). Through play, children socialize with peers and adults, develop autonomy, create emotional attachment to places, acquire physical and social skills, and build themselves as citizens.

Social class is an important variable to understand how children enjoy the city. Previous studies show that children from middle and upper classes are more subjected to hyper-protection and institutionalization processes (Leverett, 2011; Sarmento, 2018), while children from lower classes represent an *outdoor childhood* (Karsten, 2005) and are, therefore, more likely to use public spaces (Pinto and Bichara, 2017; Araújo, 2019). However, the former, due to their economic and cultural capital, can take 'better' advantage of all the city's many opportunities.

In this pandemic, children's use of public spaces and outdoor activities have been drastically reduced, and under lockdown almost all their time was spent indoors. Children and their families had to adapt to a new reality of mitigation measures. For children, some consequences of the pandemic are increased time spent online and playing videogames (SICAD, 2020), social isolation, and various impacts on their development and physical and emotional health (Kyriazis et al, 2020; Russel and Stenning, 2020; United Nations, 2020). In Portugal during lockdown, the government authorized the 'short hygienic walk', unlike other European countries such as Spain. However, in

Porto, parks were closed and these brief walks were meant for getting fresh air and exercise, and thus excluded children's free play and other uses of public spaces.

The COVID-19 virus's spread across our globalized world exposed the paradoxes and flaws of neoliberal societies and initiated multiple transformations in the uses of public spaces and in urban childhood. The pandemic revealed social and economic inequalities in cities, and vulnerable groups were the most affected (Berkowitz et al, 2020; Biglieri et al, 2020; United Nations, 2020), among them children and, in particular, children from lower-class families and also children with disabilities:

> Moreover, the harmful effects of this pandemic will not be distributed equally. They are expected to be most damaging for children in the poorest countries, and in the poorest neighbourhoods, and for those in already disadvantaged or vulnerable situations. (United Nations, 2020: 2)

Methodological approach

Our research is based on an ethnographic study of children's use of public spaces. The study gave us a deeper understanding of the practices of children in urban parks, particularly in playgrounds, and of class and cultural dynamics. Ethnographic fieldwork involving participant and non-participant observation occurred during the spring and summer of 2019 and of 2020. We observed two parks (Pasteleira and Covelo) using the same evaluative matrix before the outbreak and post-lockdown. We assessed variables such as gender; age; children's preferred place(s); interaction with peers and adults; children's ownership of space; and factors related to adult supervision (who, what kind). After the lockdown, observations were carried out twice a week in each park and lasted about two hours; the children observed were between two and 12 years old.

Participatory drawings and focus group activities also occurred with children in two institutions (a private school and a social center). To query children's parents/guardians on their lockdown experiences and the pandemic's effects on children's park use and their daily lives, we carried out 30 semi-structured interviews in the parks with adults selected from our observation itinerary. Social class, an important variable in our research, was evaluated on the basis of collected information regarding the children's neighborhood and the educational institution they attended, as well as parents' academic qualifications, performed jobs, and professional status. Children's participation in research has specific methodological and ethical issues (Morrow and Richards, 1996; Christensen, 2004) related to assuring that children understand the objectives of the research and the implications of their participation and, further, that they consent to participate (to be also provided by their responsible adults). Following international guidelines for sociological research, the confidentiality and anonymity of participants were assured by making all children's names and image confidential. The potential impacts of the research on children and to share findings with them were also considered. During the focus groups, findings were presented to children and they were invited to express their views.

Away from the park in lockdown and returning after to live a 'new normal'

As stated, the region of Porto was the pandemic's initial epicenter in Portugal, enduring a 47-day lockdown. Mitigation measures included closing schools and encouraging people to study and work from home. To go out was not allowed, except to buy basic goods and a once-daily brief walk for adults and children. Our interviews with adults in the parks show that, for younger children, lockdown was very stressful, as they missed outdoor activities, for example going to the parks, and many did not understand why they could not go out. A father of four children stated:

> 'They missed the park a lot. We used to come here every day as their school is very near. The smaller ones didn't know what was going on. It was not easy.' (Father, Pasteleira park, July 7, 2020)

However, for most of the older children, the lockdown was not felt as an imprisonment, as even before the pandemic they preferred to stay home to 'play online' (use the internet and videogames). For them, lockdown was an opportunity to do this without their parents' disapproval since the latter had to work or had no other way to occupy the children's spare time.

In order to keep their children entertained, many parents, in both parks and from different social classes, told us that they started to let their children (up to two or three years old) play online. The grandparents of a three-year-old girl reported:

> 'Her parents had to work at home and she kept asking for their attention. To keep her occupied, they started letting her play on the cell phone. Now they are trying to get her to stop because they don't think it's healthy for a child.' (Grandparents, Covelo park, July 4, 2020)

This is consistent with data showing that internet and videogame use by children and teenagers has significantly increased with the lockdown (SICAD, 2020), and it is nowadays considered one of the most unsettling challenges to parents and to the wider society.

Turning to the analyzed parks, Covelo park is located in a central area inhabited mostly by middle- and upper-middle-class families. With no other green spaces around, the park is busy every day, and the playground is the most vibrant area visited by people of different ages. Pasteleira park is found in the city's

children interacting with others outside their group and sharing objects they had brought from home, mostly beach buckets and shovels. Although some parents may not feel comfortable with this, most of them assumed it was difficult to avoid it:

> 'In relation to that [sharing objects], there's nothing we can do. We just have to clean the objects afterwards and their [children's] hands.' (Mother, Covelo park, July 30, 2020)

It was also in the sandbox that we observed more interaction between mothers who did not know each other. The interaction between children also encouraged social interaction between parents.

Conclusion

As stated by Hall (1990), distances are recreated within socio-cultural categories. The pandemic radically changed the dominant perceptions of legitimate or desirable proximity and distance, in line with previous trends of social hygienization and securitization (Reigner, 2016). This particularly affects groups with less power, such as children.

Children's play before and post-lockdown varies according to age, social class, and ethnicity. One very important finding of this research relates to age differences: younger children do not understand social distance and still play free from these concerns, using the parks and interacting with other children as they did before the lockdown. These practices also stimulate social interactions between their parents and other caregivers. However, social pressure over older children (age five+) increases, and some families do not even let their children use the parks' playgrounds. Our research findings point clearly to a more solitary play in public parks, mostly promoted by parents and caregivers. We wonder if the public parks are becoming a kind of 'alternative backyard' instead of public spaces characterized by the possibility of encounter with the *other*, the *unexpected*, the *different*.

The psychological and social impacts of the pandemic for children are yet to be evaluated, but we already observe that social and urban inequalities continue to intensify in the COVID-19 crisis, even after lockdown. Children are actors who need to play and be with others beyond the social realm of their families as part of their growth as individuals with rights to the city.

Public policy should look urgently into these issues and try to find reasonable solutions to the lack of children's voices in urban and public space planning. Decision makers should rethink urban planning policies in light of what the pandemic has taught us: the importance of the streets as spaces for walking, playing, and for intergenerational and cross-cultural socialization; the urgency of creating more green spaces for the well-being of the communities; acknowledging that the periphery and the most vulnerable groups are the ones who suffer more from urban inequalities; and finally, a change in paradigms where children and their right to the city are at the center of urban planning.

Acknowledgements

This work was supported by Fundação para a Ciência e a Tecnologia, I.P., under the Project PTDC/SOC-SOC/30415/2017.

References

Araújo, M.J. (2019) 'Brincar no bairro: descobrir o lazer no tempo livre através da sociabilidade nos espaços de logradouro', in M. J. Araújo et al (eds) *InfantiCidades: pelo direito a brincar*. Porto: Escola Superior de Educação, pp 23–46.

Berkowitz, R.L., Gao, X., Michaels, E.K. and Mujahid, M.S. (2020) 'Structurally vulnerable neighbourhood environments and racial/ethnic COVID-19 inequities'. *Cities & Health*, DOI: 10.1080/23748834.2020.1792069

Biglieri, S., Vidovich, L. and Keil, R. (2020) 'City as the core of contagion? Repositioning COVID-19 at the social and spatial periphery of urban society'. *Cities & Health*, DOI: 10.1080/23748834.2020.1788320

Christensen, P.H. (2004) Children's participation in ethnographic research: issues of power and representation. *Children & Society*, 18(2): 165–76.

Hall, E.T. (1990) *The Hidden Dimension*. New York: Anchor Books.

Farné, R. (2017) 'Play and the city'. *Journal of Theories and Research in Education*, 12(1).

Fyhri, A., Hjorthol, R. Mackett, R.L., Nordgaard Fortel, T. and Kyttä, M. (2011) 'Children's active travel and independent mobility in four countries: development, social contributing trends and measures'. *Transport Policy*, 18: 703–10.

Karsten, L. (2005) 'It all used to be better? Different generations on continuity and change in urban children's daily use of space'. *Children's Geographies*, 3, 275–90.

Kyriazis, A., Mews G., Belpaire, E., Aerts, J. and Malik, S.A. (2020) 'Physical distancing, children and urban health: the COVID-19 crisis' impact on children and how this could affect future urban planning and design policies'. *Cities & Health*, DOI: 10.1080/23748834.2020.1809787

Lefebvre, H. (1968) *Le droit à la ville*. Paris: Anthropos.

Leverett, S. (2011) 'Children's spaces', in P. Foley and S. Leverett (eds) *Children and Young People's Spaces*. Basingstoke: Palgrave Macmillan, pp 9–24.

Morrow, V. and Richards, M. (1996) The ethics of social research with children: an overview. *Children & Society*, 10(2): 90–105.

Pinto, P. and Bichara, I. (2017) 'O que dizem as crianças sobre os espaços públicos onde brincam'. *Interação em Psicologia*, 21(1): 28–38.

Rasmussen, K. (2004) 'Places for children: children's places'. *Childhood: A Global Journal of Child Research*, 11(2): 155–74.

Reigner, H. (2016) *Neoliberal Rationality and Neohygienist Morality: A Foucaldian Analysis of Safe and Sustainable Urban Transport Policies in France*. UK: Territory, Politics, Governance.

Russel, W. and Stenning, A. (2020) 'Beyond active travel: children, play and community on streets during and after the coronavirus lockdown'. *Cities & Health*, DOI: 10.1080/23748834.2020.1795386

Sarmento, M. (2018) 'Infância e cidade: restrições e possibilidades'. *Educação*, 41(2): 232–40.

Shaw, B., Bicket, M., Elliot, B., Fagan-Watson, B., Mocca, E. and Hillman, M. (2015) *Children's Independent Mobility: An International Comparison and Recommendations for Action*. London: Report for Policy Studies Institute, University of Westminster.

SICAD (Serviço de Intervenção nos Comportamentos Aditivos e nas Dependências) (2020) *Comportamentos aditivos em tempos de COVID 19: internet e videojogos*. Retrieved from: www.sicad.pt/ BK/EstatisticaInvestigacao/EstudosConcluidos/Lists/SICAD_ ESTUDOS/Attachments/210/comportamentos%20aditivos%20 em%20tempos%20de%20COVID%20-%20Internet%20e%20 Videojogos.pdf

Tonucci, F. (2001) *La ciudad de los ninõs: un modo nuevo de pensar la ciudad*. Madrid: Fund, German Sanchez Ruiperez.

United Nations (2020) *Policy brief: The Impact of COVID-19 on Children*. Retrieved from: https://unsdg.un.org/resources/ policy-brief-impact-COVID-19-children

However, very little has been discussed in relation to the public spaces which play an implicit yet critical role in the quality of everyday life in Indian cities. At a superficial level, everyday life in public spaces involves ordinary experiences and routines that are taken for granted (Upton, 2002; Sandywell, 2004; Rajendran, 2016). This chapter is developed in the form of a think piece to highlight how examining these 'mundane' spaces and the activities performed in those spaces can provide an interesting lens to understand the altering socio-spatial relations and its impact on people's behavioral practices in the pandemic and post-pandemic context. The discussions are mainly drawn upon from a pilot study employing participant observation and photo documentation methods to understand the impacts of COVID-19 on the everyday public spaces in Chennai city, capital of Tamil Nadu, India.

Public spaces and everyday life in Indian cities

Everyday public spaces in India evoke diverse experiences as being noisy, congested, vibrant, robust, busy, and lively. These qualities manifest themselves physically and provide a multi-layered structuring of the urban spaces that is organic, multi-functional, and fluid in nature. The very reason why often for a visitor these places are seemingly chaotic, but for a native they embed an inherent order, one which is organically developed through spatial practice, occupation, and negotiation overtime. Studying these complex urban settings and practices using the everyday lens offers a 'rich repository of urban meaning' (Crawford, 2008) and facilitates towards comprehending their spatial manifestation and underlying patterns of behavior.

One significant place/space typology which manifests the rich and complex nature of everyday life in public spaces in India are the streets (Tandon and Sehgal, 2017). The everyday life in streets provides interesting cues for deciphering the 'urban experience and social needs which are more than mere conceptual abstractions' (Stevens, 2007: 7). The very diverse qualities and character of these streets and the meanings they might have for those who live it, and in particular the complex tensions which arise between different needs, different meanings, and different users in space (Stevens, 2007) can facilitate the unraveling of the various factors that embed the matrix of everyday life.

Indian city streets are multifunctional and have traditionally served as key public spaces (Brower, 1996; Carr, 1992), around which social life has revolved hence can be considered an essential public space typology (Deore and Lathia, 2019). They provide the means for/to access, it is a zone where most of the daily activity takes place be it the morning walks and commercial activity of the street vendors. And for people who buy from these roadside shops, it is also the parking area for their two-wheeler and, in some cases the shops sprawl and encroach into the pavement/streets interrupting the very basic faction of movement of the people/vehicles. The intertwined and informal nature of transactions, behavioral patterns, functions, and spatial structuring can be cited as the main reason why adopting/adapting to the social distancing in these spaces was extremely challenging.

Case study and methodology

The state of Tamil Nadu is famously called the Land of temples, and Chennai city, the capital of the state, is a typical example which has many Hindu temples in its urban landscape. The public spaces chosen for this pilot study are around the 8th century Sri Parthasarathy temple complex dedicated to Lord Krishna located at Thiruvellikeni, Chennai. Deriving its name from the holy tank, Thiru-alli-keni (Sacred Lily Pond, in Tamil) neighborhood is inseparable from the temple context. The streets and the other public spaces surrounding the temple support several retail activities and particularly the informal sector of the city. The weekly street markets, especially when it falls on auspicious days, brings people from the across the city. These markets are a major attraction as they offer a variety of items catering to all age groups, from toys to household utensils at reasonable prices. Apart from this, the market is especially popular for its additional entertainment activities such as balloon shooting, 'robot' astrology, and handicraft making, adding more vibrancy to the overall experiences of the neighborhood.

The study adopted visual research methods employing participant observation and observational walking (Pierce and Lawhon, 2015) during the lockdown phase to gather data for understanding the multi-dimensional role of public spaces and people's engagement as well as their relationship with community and public space use during pandemic situations. Using the lens of everyday life, a comparative analysis of the socio-spatial practices in the public spaces before and after lockdown was conducted. The key observations and reflections from the analysis are summarized thematically.

Social distancing versus place engagement

One of the visible changes caused by the impact of COVID-19 on city life globally is the social distancing in public spaces, making it an urban phenomenon that has altered the perspective of planning and design of city spaces. In the public spaces around the temple, the concept of social distancing and its transgression needs to be approached from a socio-cultural perspective as people's place engagement and activities are embedded in an organic and informal urban matrix with deeper meanings and connotations.

The public spaces outside the temple serve as an informal and flexible setting accommodating hawkers, short-term parking, and provide opportunities for spontaneous and casual social interactions, and a vibrant place experience. Often everyday public spaces are valorized as sites of spontaneity, and the lived experiences in such spaces possess deep-rooted meanings which are often implicit, but when explored carefully may reveal interesting concepts towards place engagement in cities. The public spaces around the temple can be seen largely as loose (Franck and Stevens, 2006) or incidental spaces (Rajendran, 2016) spaces whose functional use is rather fluid in nature and allows 'people to recognise the possibilities inherent and make use of those possibilities for their own ends, facing the potential risks of doing so' (Franck and Stevens, 2006: 2). These spaces play a vital role in providing opportunities for enacting place appropriation, embodied spatial practices, and engagement with places. Such opportunities are an inherent need for developing and negotiating one's identity and belonging in places (Rajendran et al, 2014; Rajendran, 2016). Linked strongly to the temple context, the tangible aspects of the public marketplace, people, objects and colors create an engaging place experience for the residents, enabling a strong sense of identity both at an individual and collective level.

Such public spaces implore to be viewed and understood as a part of larger social–cultural ecosystem of cities to effectively implement strategies for pandemic control measures. Figures 14.1 and 14.2 clearly show there is little differences in terms of physical distancing during social interaction and transactional activities with the vendors, and it is challenging to regulate activities and impose measures of social distancing using a top-down approach.

Spatial structures of public spaces

The market streets are bordered by the temple wall on one side and the traditional row housing settlement on the other side. The activities in these streets are more structured due to the linear spatial arrangement, and the absence of informal vendors during the lockdown created deserted streets. The impact of the phased approach (shop closures on certain days and times) to lockdown on the diverse public spaces (streets, transitions spaces, mixed use spaces) around the temple was also dependent on the spatial structure of these spaces. The

Figure 14.1: Public spaces outside Parthasarathy Temple (Chennai, India) before lockdown

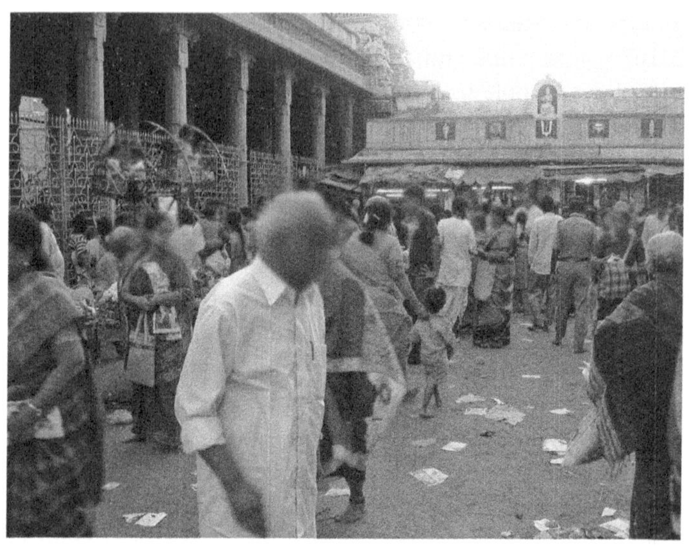

Source: Lakshmi Priya Rajendran

lockdown measures were easier to implement in a more linear market street space as the movement and interaction of people were considerably reduced once the hawkers were restricted to use the spaces. Imposing restrictions was relatively challenging outside the temple areas as the activities and the spatial arrangement were more fluid. Also with people being allowed to visit temples this required associated small vendors and shops (flower shops, ritual things shops, and so on) to be operational (see Figures 14.3 and 14.4).

Informal sectors and public space

The impact of lockdown on the dynamic and multifunctional nature of public spaces around the temple can potentially alter on one hand, the relationships of activities and people – the

Figure 14.2: Public spaces outside Parthasarathy Temple (Chennai, India) after lockdown

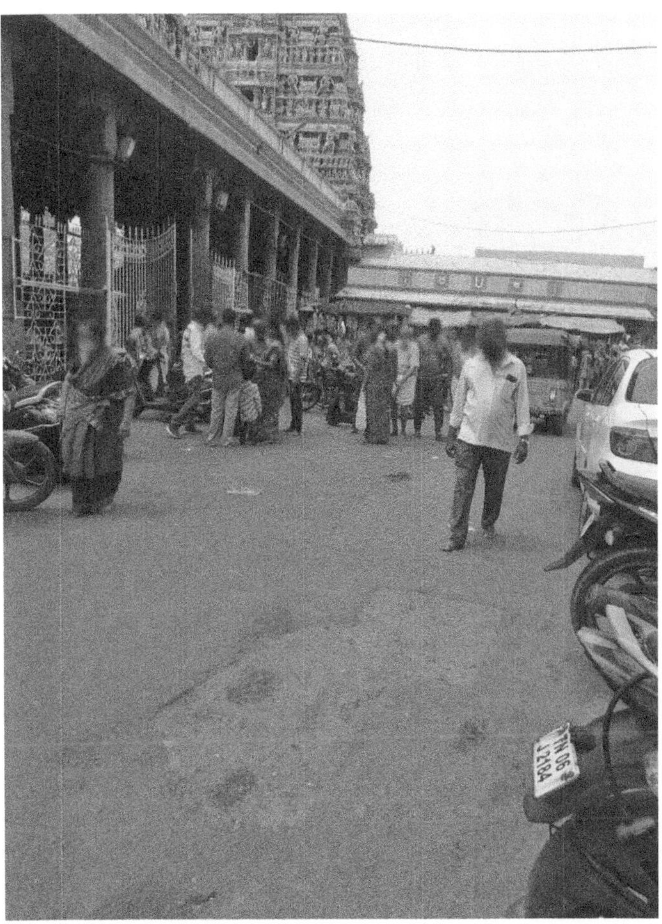

Source: Lakshmi Priya Rajendran

process of interaction, engagement, and transaction, and on the other hand, the spatial pattern and structure of the public space that are implicit (affordances, flexibility) and explicit (circulation, access). Such alterations at different scales are

Figure 14.3: Street spaces used by local vendors (Chennai, India) before lockdown

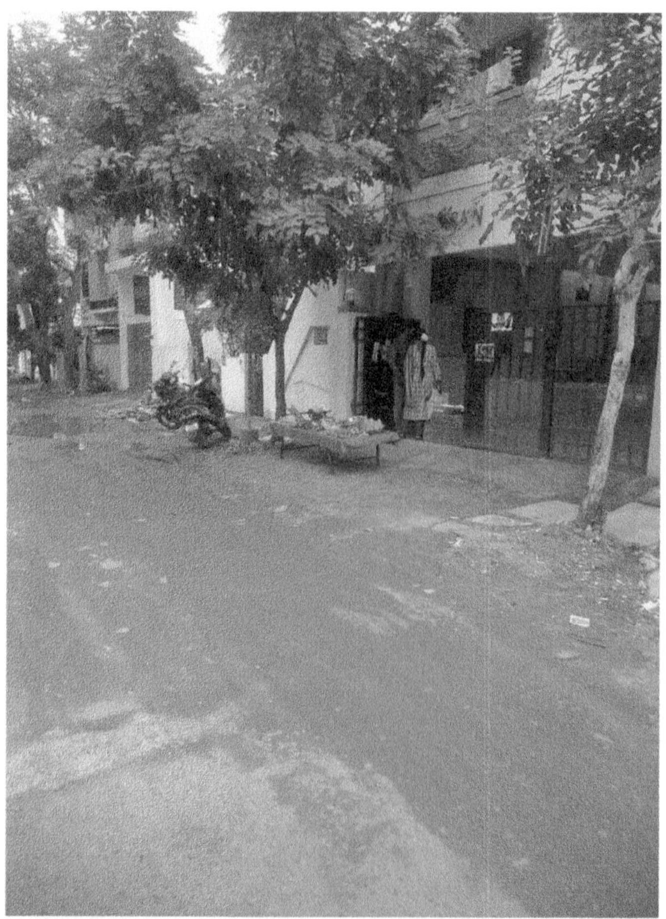

Source: Lakshmi Priya Rajendran

experienced differently by different user groups. For instance, street vendors and hawkers who occupy transitional spaces, spaces like boundaries and entry points of the temple, face a significant impact on their livelihood due to reduced sales, especially when dealing with perishable goods (fruits,

Figure 14.4: Street spaces used by local vendors (Chennai, India) after lockdown

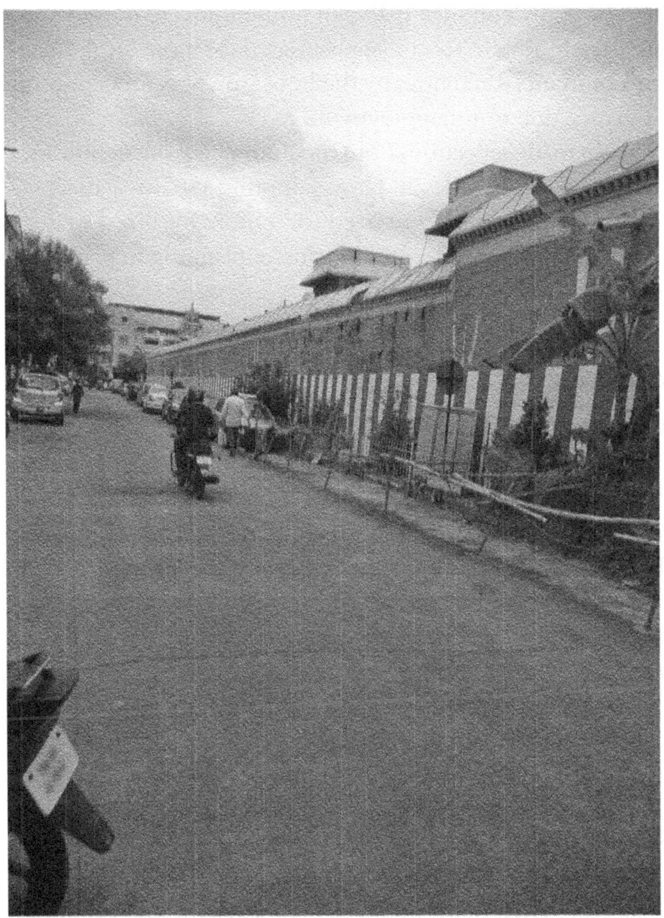

Source: Lakshmi Priya Rajendran

vegetables, flowers, fast food, street food, and so on). A relatively more organized business of small vendors within and near areas of the public places experience poor or no turnout of their regular customers, which affects their business in the mid- and long-term. Interestingly there has also been some local creative spatial response to the impact of the lockdown whereby many entrance spaces of households are transformed into 'private-public' spaces, appropriated for more local, small-scale commercial activities by the house-owners for economic sustenance due to unemployment.

The thematic reflections from the study show the significance of public spaces in cities and how adopting a socio-spatial perspective brings to light the need for a more localized strategy and approach for effective and inclusive planning in pandemic and post-pandemic contexts.

Conclusion

Moving away and zooming out from the street scale to a neighborhood and city scale, we see that everyday public spaces, often viewed as 'mundane', provide a matrix for people to operate the concepts of identity, belonging, and equity in cities. The interrelated dynamics of society and space (Netto, 2017) is manifested through corporeal performative practices enacted within the informal urban structures of public spaces in Indian cities. These urban spaces which allow for significant socio-spatial relationships to merge are unfortunately overlooked as 'spatiality tends to be peripheralised into the background as reflection, container, stage, environment, or external constraint of human behaviour and social action' (Proshansky et al, 1970; Soja 1996: 71).

As the famous landmarks of Indian cities remain deserted, public spaces that deliver the essential services, street vendors, and corner shops still see people negotiating/adhering/transgressing the spatial rules imposed during the lockdown. It is important to acknowledge that the everyday urbanism in cities has the potential to implicitly define socio-spatial behavior and patterns, and to review the existing public spaces and the role it can potentially play in the future to make cities liveable, and valuable lessons should be taken forward by architects, planners, and urban designers.

Post-pandemic, it will be interesting to see how people re-engage with public spaces making new trajectories to examine public spaces as enablers of socio-cultural resilience in cities. While people are engaging with newer medium and means of interaction/encounters (both physical and digital),the lockdown phase has nevertheless thrown light on the significance of the mundane yet multi-layered and (extra)ordinary everyday spaces in cities.

References

Brower, S. (1996) *Good Neighborhoods*. Westport, CT: Praeger.

Carr, S. (1992) *Public Space*. Cambridge and New York: Cambridge University Press.

Crawford, M. (2008) 'Introduction', in J. Chase, M. Crawford and J. Kaliski (eds) *Everyday Urbanism*. New York: Monacelli Press.Deore, P. and Lathia, S. (2019) 'Streets as public spaces: lessons from street vending in Ahmedabad, India'. *Urban Planning*, 4(2): 138–53.

Franck, K. and Stevens, Q. (2006) *Loose Space: Possibility and Diversity in Urban Life*. Abingdon/New York: Routledge.

Netto, V.M. (2017) *The Social Fabric of Cities*. Abingdon/New York: Routledge.

Pierce, J. and Lawhon, M. (2015) 'Walking as method: toward methodological forthrightness and comparability in urban geographical research'. *The Professional Geographer*, 67(4): 655–62.

Proshansky, H.M., Ittelson, W.H. and Rivlin, L.G. (1970) 'The influence of the physical environment on behavior: some basic assumptions', in *Environmental Psychology: Man and His Physical Setting*. Toronto: Holt, Rinehart and Winston.

Rajendran, L.P. (2016) 'Understanding identity and belonging through incidental spaces'. *Proceedings of the Institution of Civil Engineers – Urban Design and Planning*, 169(4): 165–74.

time, they have demonstrated their resilience with an ability to self-sustain and through their various, critical roles supporting the community. Given that informal sectors have usually been considered problematic and treated unequally by the government, the experiences and initiatives of street vendors during the pandemic in Hanoi represent a form of local resilience that deserves a closer look in our work to understand and minimize urban inequality.

This chapter examines the informal livelihoods of street vendors in Hanoi, Vietnam during the COVID-19 crisis, highlighting their initiatives (employed amid public health restrictions) to generate income and provide affordable foods and critical services to others, especially low-income families (see also Volume 1, Chapter Two). We analyze data from local reports and 22 interviews with street vendors conducted in April 2020, to illuminate the survival strategies and adaptive capacity of the urban poor in Hanoi. This sheds light on the role of social capital in enhancing resilience, through community collaboration, sharing, and solidarity. Given social capital has multiple meanings and applications, this chapter refers to the capability of people to work together for mutual objectives through personal connection, communal network, and virtual platforms in societies (Burt, 1992; Ellison et al, 2007). Street vendors' practices during the lockdown in Hanoi aligns with Fukuyama (1995), who defines social capital as the presence of a certain set of informal values or norms shared among local residents that enable collaboration and bonding; both are significant in building resilience (Agnitsch et al, 2006).

Informal livelihoods and COVID-19 crisis in Hanoi

Residents in Hanoi have a long tradition of running small-scale and informal businesses to mitigate their lack of formal employment or social security programs (Pasquier-Doumer et al, 2017). To many, public sector work is out of reach and/or low-paid. Better-paid private sector employment requires specific qualifications and time commitments inconsistent with work-life balance. Therefore, informal livelihoods are the primary option to generate either main income for low-skilled workers or extra income for low-paid state employees (key players in the informal economy).

More than just earning their livelihoods, informal workers offer affordable goods and services to the general population, especially the urban poor. They connect farmers and small-scale manufacturers in the periphery to inner-city consumers. Goods – especially fresh food, household items, and clothes – are obtained directly from producers and sold to consumers with minimal transaction fees imposed by informal workers. Providers of services, such as barbers, motorbike repairers, and locksmiths, are also widely found on Hanoi's streets; further, the stalls and carts of local food and tea merchants serve as community eating areas, helping to ensure a vibrant street life.

The adverse impacts of COVID-19 have created unprecedented challenges for informal workers. The most effective and widespread measure the government has employed to contain the virus has been strictly enforced lockdown of communities. Social distancing rules and gathering prohibitions temporarily eliminate public space use rights for most residents including street vendors, now forced to stop their income-generating activities. During the lockdown in Hanoi, from March 28 to April 23, using public space for informal trading was not allowed. Most residents, particularly low-income families, lost access to affordable foods and services while, goods, especially perishables, were stuck with farmers. From August 17 to September 5, social distancing policies were reinstated to ban public gathering and the operation of non-essential businesses in public spaces.

Government responses

In early April 2020, Hanoi People's Committee conducted a survey to understand the impact of COVID-19 on local residents (RISED, 2020). While the survey's results are still confidential, they are expected to help the government enact an effective economic growth plan during and after the pandemic. The survey targeted three population groups: 1) local residents of Hanoi; 2) school and university students; and 3) workers and family-based manufacturers and retailers. Notably, no specific concern was given to informal workers, whose lives depend on being able to work in public space. It appears that these 'official' government actors failed to recognize their important role in the city's economy likely led to informal workers' (for example street vendors) exclusion from the survey.

At the end of April 2020, the Vietnamese government announced Decision No15/2020/QD/TTg to implement a 62 trillion VND (approximately 2.6 billion USD) aid program for residents impacted by COVID-19. Six groups of residents can apply for this financial support. Almost all of these come from formal economic sectors. Residents whose incomes come from informal sectors, such as street vendors, traders, and service providers are listed as a subgroup within this policy. However, eligible applicants must verify their residential status and/or recent business activities when applying to the local authority. These conditions marginalize informal workers who are often immigrants and/or lack fixed addresses or places of work. This suggests a lack of policy infrastructure to support informal economies under crises such as those imposed by COVID-19.

Local resilience and survival initiatives

During lockdown, Hanoi's street vendors and residents devised a range of survival *tactics*, to borrow the term coined by de Certeau (1984: 30), in response to lockdown *strategies* imposed by the government. Although these initiatives are very diverse, they share some qualities that reveal the role of local social capital practices of community sharing and solidarity.

Embracing solidarity through grassroots community organizations

While local governments still struggle to financially support informal workers, community-based groups have quickly materialized to aid the urban poor. For instance, ATM stations introduced in mid-April by generous individuals to dispense free rice, were welcomed by many poor workers (donated rice is packed and distributed by volunteers). These ATMs, organized by local authorities, provide shelters and instructions for rice gatherers to socially distance. A practice now widely adopted by various other communities, semi-automatic rice dispensers (made with donated materials by tech students) are programmed to give three free kilograms of rice per person per day.

Mrs B, a trash collector and a mother of two, claims the free rice helps her family to survive for a week (Interview, April 2020). She does not know how to apply for support from the government because she is an unregistered resident and itinerant worker. Her husband, an intermittent hotel security guard, has not been paid for months. While Mrs B appreciates the free food from local community groups and rent reduction from her landlord, lacking support amid the precarious economics brought on by COVID-19 led her to reduce the family's already modestly portioned meals.

Solidarity, demonstrated through giving, sharing, and caring, led by grassroots organizations, and facilitated by local authorities, provides critically important relief to the poor and the government. During the crisis, 'a little bite when hungry is worth a feast when full' (interview with Mr H, a rice donor, in April 2020).

Shifting to mobile trading

During the March–April lockdown, when informal pop-up stalls and outdoor markets were closed, footpath traders quickly

and assisting disadvantaged workers from formal sectors, urban inequality will remain rampant so long as the vital role of informal economies is underestimated. However, local governments and neighborhood-level community groups have been flexibly supportive to poor residents, especially informal street vendors and service providers, who are popular yet lack legitimacy in the official policy frameworks of Vietnam's municipal and state governments.

This chapter highlights how informal economies, including those newly established through ICT, have managed to survive in light of COVID-19's impacts. Through their *tactics*, informal workers have maintained their urban livelihoods and provided alternative economic opportunities to residents struggling with the government's lockdown *strategies*.

The stories discussed in this chapter have implications. In cities such as Hanoi, where the coexistence of formality and informality have always shaped urban economies and wider society, the pandemic and strictly enforced reactionary measures demonstrate informal sectors' resilience and their role in softening various economic and social impacts. This resilience together with the sense of solidarity brought by individual, community, and local government initiatives represent a form of social capital essential for supporting disadvantaged residents. Given COVID-19 is unpredictable – Hanoi reapplied the social distancing policies from August 17 to September 5 (the time this chapter was being written) – the question is: to what extent can social capital help the urban poor deal with impacts of this and future pandemics? Indeed, it is important, in the long term, to enact policies that better recognize the significance of informal economies and workers to urban livelihoods. This in turn would help governments mitigate urban inequality via effective, progressive policies and programs to identify and assist the most vulnerable during these public health and economic lockdowns.

References

Agnitsch, K., Flora, J. and Ryan, V. (2006) 'Bonding and bridging social capital: the interactive effects on community action'. *Community Development*, 37(1): 36–51.

Burt, R. (1992) *Structural Holes: The Social Structure of Competition*. Cambridge: Harvard University Press.

de Certeau, M. (1984) *The Practice of Everyday Life*. Berkeley: University of California Press.

Decision, No15/2020/QD/TTg (2020) *Implementation of Financial Aid Program for Local Residents Suffering from Covid-19*, Vietnamese Government Office (in Vietnamese).

Ellison, N., Steinfield, C. and Lampe, C. (2007) 'The benefits of Facebook friends: social capital and college students' use of online social network sites'. *Journal of Computer-Mediated Communication*, 12(4): 1143–68.

Fukuyama, F. (1995) *Trust: The Social Virtues and the Creation of Prosperity*. London: Hamish Hamilton.

International Labour Organization (ILO) (2020) *ILO Brief: COVID-19 Crisis and The Informal Economy*. Geneva: ILO.

Pasquier-Doumer, L., Oudin, X. and Thang, N. (2017) *The Importance of Household Businesses and the Informal Sector for Inclusive Growth in Vietnam and the Informal Sector*. Hanoi: The Gioi Publisher.

Pollack, T. et al (2020) 'Emerging COVID-19 success story: Vietnam's commitment to containment', in *Exemplars in Global Health*. Retrieved from: https://ourworldindata.org/covid-exemplar-vietnam

RISED (2020) *Survey Questionnaires on the Impact of Covid 19 on Residents in Hanoi*. The Institute of Research and Socio-Economic Development. Retrieved from: http://rised.org.vn/

Thai, H.M.H., Khuat, H.T. and Kim, H.M. (2021) 'Urban form, the use of ICT and smart cities in Vietnam', in H.M. Kim, S. Sabri and A. Kent (eds) *Smart Cities for Technological and Social Innovation*. Amsterdam: Elsevier, pp 137–56.

Wertheim-Heck, S. (2020) *The Impact of the COVID-19 Lockdown on the Diets of Hanoi's Urban Poor*. International Institute for Environment and Development. Retrieved from: www.iied.org/impact-COVID-19-lockdown-diets-hanois-urban-poor

PART III

Public Space and Mobility

jaws of motor vehicles – including the car but also the float planes typically roaring over its tree canopy and carbon thirsty passenger jets shaking the skies above – Stanley Park almost seemed to revert back to a more primeval, unadulterated version of itself protected from human pollution.

Stanley Park's transformation from noisy car park to resurgent nature was a common story after COVID-19, which precipitated both a global surge in cycling and noticing nature (see also Volume 4, Chapter Four). It was a strange, ironic rupture: one ecological catastrophe (COVID-19, a zoonotic disease) pressing pause on another (the system of automobility). Stanley Park's transformation did not last long – the motor vehicle returned in late June to half its former road space, and then all of it by late September when new dedicated space for cycling was fully removed – and the cycling surge has failed to put a dent in greenhouse gas emissions (GHGs). Far worse, it could well be succeeded by the ecological calamity of expanded car use, causing more deaths than COVID-19, as people recoil from busy sidewalks, eschew public transit, purchase their first cars, and flood the suburban real estate market. Of the two blades in COVID-19's double-edged sword for cycling, automobility's expansion threatens a longer, deeper cut.

On the bright side, the pandemic accomplished something extraordinary: it proved that transport behavior is not as difficult to change as people had assumed, and 'society can reconfigure to less car dependent lifestyles' (Marsden et al, 2020: 90). As if overnight, COVID-19 demonstrated – even in Canada, one of the most privileged, fossil energy intensive nations in the world (with the highest GHG emissions per capita in the G20) – that urban car dependence is not a *fait accompli*, but rather a social and political construct embedded in our built environments, one that people can, if push comes to shove, disassemble. COVID-19 also showed that, even Canadians, in spite of their extreme car-dependence, can cycle instead – if they enjoy access to safe, connected spaces to do so, which many do not.

Drawing on Canadian cases, this chapter asks: will the pandemic lead to an expanded cycling city, or will the car reap the rewards of disruption? And what sort of cycling will emerge after COVID-19? How can cities use cycling as a tool for interspecies mobility justice, by making space for the voices, capabilities, and knowledges of marginalized and colonized persons (Sheller, 2018), including other-than-human persons and habitats (Scott, 2020a)?

To explore these questions, I draw on field observations of cycling under COVID-19 collected during spring and summer of 2020 in Vancouver and Halifax, as well as data from a larger ethnographic study on city cycling undertaken before the pandemic (2014–18) (Scott, 2020b). In what follows, I examine one prominent way in which Canadian cities, while elaborating lockdown measures and physical distancing rules, sought quickly to accommodate active mobilities at the expense of the car, so-called Slow Streets. I then broaden my lens to consider how cycling after COVID-19 might expand into the vast auto-burbs sprawling far beyond the pale of the urban cores where Slow Streets and bike lanes reside.

Slow Streets for whom?

The sociality on Beach Avenue lit up after the City of Vancouver turned it into a massive bike lane (see Figure 16.1). A day after Vancouver removed cars from Stanley Park, it turned half of Beach Avenue, a busy four-lane arterial highway approaching the park, into dedicated cycling space using pylons. Thousands of people cycling poured into Beach Avenue every day, many of whom were recreational rather than commuter cyclists, all of whom had never enjoyed such ample time and space for riding this oceanic street. The street's atmosphere instantly became more festive, removed from the threat of violent encounters with motor vehicles. Whereas the successful Stanley Park experiment, unfortunately, did not last – the (democratically elected) Vancouver Park Board capitulated with irate motorists

Figure 16.1: Sociality on Beach Avenue, Vancouver

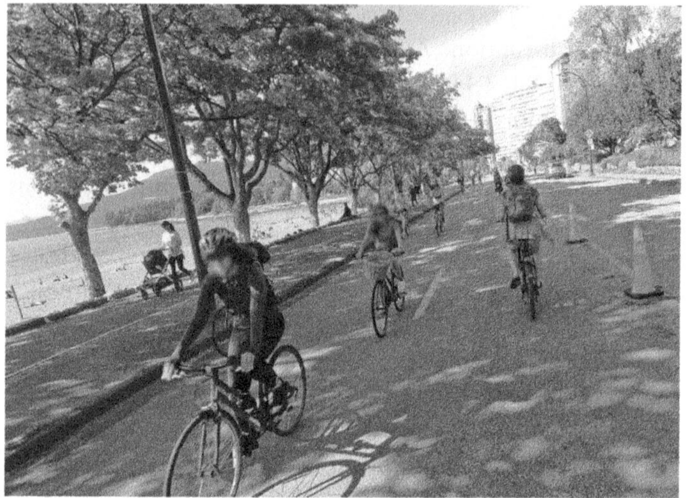

Source: Nicholas A. Scott

promising 'war' on social media if cars and car-based businesses were not allowed back in – the new Beach Avenue persists (as of time of writing, October 2020). Together, they revealed extraordinary latent demand for cycling.

The global surge in cycling after COVID-19 helped move many cities to initiate and accelerate off-car transitions. Following the lead of Milan, Paris, Bogotá, and Oakland, some cities in Canada sought to surf on the novel COVID-19 toward sustainable transport by creating networks of streets that restrict access to, and slow down, the car (generally a politically toxic move in Canada, as evidenced by the backlash against Stanley Park's car closure). Vancouver and Halifax, notably, rapidly assembled Slow Streets in their core neighborhoods, which deploy rudimentary roadblocks to exclude non-local traffic (save delivery vehicles) and limit local cars to 30km/hr (a critical threshold for preventing cars from killing cyclists and pedestrians in collisions). After transforming Beach Avenue, Vancouver built out by summer a 50km network of

Slow Streets, building on already existing cycling infrastructure. Despite their lo-tech, DIY appearance, they proved to be wildly popular with residents. Halifax created 20 such Slow Streets, along quiet residential roads off major arteries. Intriguingly, they saw more mixed results – pointing to a useful comparison.

Slow Streets in Vancouver and Halifax faced two significant public critiques. The first critique highlights their failure to exclude fast (that is, >30km/hr) motor vehicles, their central purpose. I experienced this myself while cycling on multiple Slow Streets in both cities in summer 2020, feeling motorists blow by me after easily circumventing the roadblocks before accelerating to the next temporary barrier. Whereas in Vancouver this limitation led to calls for improving and expanding Slow Streets (Vancouver has plans to construct 170km more), in Halifax it may have helped undercut public interest in keeping them around. The City of Halifax removed their Slow Streets in September, ostensibly because of an incoming tropical storm. I suggest this divergence relates not to Vancouver's nice weather (as is often suggested) but to the fact that Vancouver's Slow Streets were superimposed on pre-existing greenways – popular cycling routes that already enjoyed (politically hard won) traffic calming measures. Halifax's Slow Streets lacked a firm foundation.

The second critique of Slow Streets is that they represent but a drop in the bucket, covering only a minuscule proportion (~2 percent) of Vancouver's and Halifax's overall road networks. As a result, Slow Streets could scarcely challenge the car and some of Canada's most salient mobility injustices, such as the anti-Black racism baked into Vancouver's and Halifax's car infrastructure. In the 1960s and 1970s, these cities bulldozed and displaced prominent urban Black communities (Hogan's Alley in Vancouver, Africville in Halifax) for new car-exclusive bridges and highways in brazen, institutionalized acts of environmental racism. To reach Black, Indigenous and other racialized populations, who are disproportionately excluded

to live in cycling-friendly central cities. If city cycling is to advance mobility justice and help extend it to other-than-human persons, it will need to contest (not further augment) the over-consumptive lifestyles of Canadians in general, and kinetic elites in particular, who have pushed the country's cities' ecological footprints and GHGs far past their ecological carrying capacities (Moore et al, 2019).

COVID-19 put the line running between exploding social inequities and ecological ruin under a spotlight. The brutal domination of some humans is intrinsically bound to that of other species by humans. Slow Streets were a good start on making a better world after the pandemic, but given the gravity of injustice the pandemic unearthed, it is time to hold cycling to a much higher standard. Cities in privileged, low-cycling nations like Canada (and the US, UK, Australia, and New Zealand) can start by building dedicated active mobility pathways and Slow Streets beyond the core into suburbs where the need is dire.

References

Ibbitson, J. (2018) 'City growth dominated by car-driving suburbs, whose votes decide elections'. *Globe*, August 20. Retrieved from: www.theglobeandmail.com/canada/article-city-growth-dominated-by-car-driving-suburbs-whose-votes-decide/

Marsden, G., Anable, J., Chatterton, T., Docherty, I., Faulconbridge, J., Murray, L., Roby, H. and Shires, J. (2020) 'Studying disruptive events: innovations in behaviour, opportunities for lower carbon transport policy?' *Transport Policy*, 94: 89–101.

Moore, J., Sussmann, C. and Rees, W.E. (2019) 'Vancouver's sustainability gap and lessons from the Southeast False Creek model sustainable community', in P. Gurstein and T.A. Hutton (eds) *Planning on the Edge: Vancouver and the Challenges of Reconciliation, Social Justice, and Sustainable Development*. Vancouver: UBC Press.

Saunders, D. (2020) 'The neighbourhood trap: the evolution of the world's inner cities has exposed a local crisis of huge proportions'. *Globe*, August 29. Retrieved from: www.theglobeandmail.com/opinion/article-the-neighbourhood-trap-the-evolution-of-the-worlds-inner-cities-has/

Scott, N.A. (2020a) 'A political theory of interspecies mobility justice'. *Mobilities*, 15(6): 880–95.

Scott, N.A. (2020b) *Assembling Moral Mobilities: Cycling, Cities & the Common Good*. Lincoln: University of Nebraska Press.

Sheller, M. (2018) *Mobility Justice: The Politics of Movement in an Age of Extremes*. New York: Verso.

SEVENTEEN

Mobility Justice and Social Inequality During the COVID-19 Pandemic in Jakarta

Harya S. Dillon and Deden Rukmana

Introduction

The first confirmed case of COVID-19 in Indonesia was reported on March 2, 2020 in Jakarta. The disease has since spread rampantly to other major cities, and Jakarta has remained to be the nation's epicenter. To flatten the epidemic curve, on March 16 Jakarta's Governor Anies Baswedan acted on President Joko Widodo's call to shelter-in-place voluntarily by restricting mobility and in particular, cutting public transportation services and limiting vehicle capacity by 50 percent. A 'soft' city-wide lockdown was imposed on April 4, effectively shutting down all schools, offices, and 'non-essential' businesses in fighting the pandemic.

After multiple two-week extensions, Mr Baswedan revealed plans to dial down the large-scale social restrictions on June 4, 2020. The two-week 'transition' period allowed some businesses to reopen in phases, keeping physical distancing measures, health and hygiene protocols, including mask-wearing mandates, and symptom surveillance. Unfortunately,

lanes are installed although not as popular to commuters. Last but not least, the Provincial Government of Jakarta is committed to keeping fares affordable by allocating subsidies. TransJakarta charges a flat fare which has not increased since 2006. With growing networks and free transfers between routes, users are actually spending less on a per-km basis.

These improvements in mobility justice run in contrast to the visible inequality in housing conditions. Jakarta has been an economic powerhouse since colonial times and, as the financial capital of Indonesia, continues to attract investments from domestic and foreign investors alike. However, poverty is still very much visible in Jakarta, especially within the informal kampung settlements surrounding modern glass towers (Prasetyanti, 2015; Salim et al, 2019). Winarso (2010) argues that Jakarta is a city of dualistic contrasts. The new suburban settlements or the 'modern' city are associated with wealth, formality, and globalized standards of urban development.

Meanwhile, the kampung city is associated with poverty, informality, and traditional standards of living. Gated communities, which house rich households who are concerned with security issues, also contributed to pockets of higher Gini indices in the suburbs. Furthermore, using a combination of location quotient and dissimilarity indices, Rukmana and Ramadhani (2020) document the pre-existing condition of inequality before the COVID-19 pandemic hit, forcing the economy to a halt.

Impacts of the pandemic on public transportation and social inequality in Jakarta

Jakarta, a megacity that is home to 9.7 million people, has been struggling with unsustainable growth of two-wheeler motorization and dwindling share of public transportation modes much like its regional peers such as Manila and Bangkok. The 2018 activity-travel diary survey found that eight in nine households (89 percent) own at least one motorcycle and that ownership is equally distributed across income levels (JICA, 2019: 39–40). The omnipresence of motorcycles offered mixed interpretations. On one hand, it signaled income growth, on the other it is choking the city. Other than the obvious congestion and air quality effects, motorcycle users often encroach on pedestrian and public spaces.

While the share of public modes has been dropping since 2002 (JICA, 2019: 56–8), it is worth noting that higher income groups are just as likely to use public transportation modes as their lower income peers. The former are more likely to use TransJakarta and urban rail systems while the latter are more inclined to use informal bus services.[1] The same survey (JICA, 2019: 37–40, 58) also found that even low-income households have access to motorcycles because of rising incomes, virtually zero down payment, and the existence of secondary markets for two-wheelers. A survey of passengers indicates that poor first/last mile connectivity, poor walkability, and the lack of convenience and comfort at transit stations are responsible for the low attractiveness of public modes (JICA, 2019: 71).

In response, the Provincial Government of Jakarta has been making great strides in improving public transportation in the last ten years. The busway systems have doubled their ridership in the past three years, and, in February 2020 achieved a major milestone of serving one million passengers per day thanks to its successful integrations with informal transit as well as its 16-years expansion and improvement of service, coupled with pedestrian improvement projects. The March 2019 launch of Jakarta's first 16km (10 miles) of MRT was hoped to reverse this decline and revitalize public transportation overall. Before the pandemic, the MRT was carrying up to 100,000 passengers per day.[2]

The pandemic hit public transportation in several ways (see also Volume 4, Chapter Sixteen). First, farebox revenue plummets since riders are now working from the safety of their homes. Overall, the MRT, TransJakarta and the state-run commuter rail service suffered a 70–90 percent drop in ridership between April and May 2020 compared to the pre-pandemic averages. Furthermore, extra spending was necessary for pandemic proofing such as hand sanitizers, thermometer guns, disinfectant sprays, and facemasks and protective gears for workers.

Second, public transportation may further suffer in the future from the cascading effect of a significantly moderated growth. Government subsidy accounts for a significant portion of public bus and MRT operations; this may get cut as the government is expected to reallocate budget for pandemic response while general revenue is shrinking. In the short run, these cuts have manifested in passengers waiting longer, which in turn may result in passengers shifting away to private modes, incurring long-term losses which may wipe out 15 years of gains in public transportation reform.

Fortunately, not all is lost. The online survey of 462 respondents conducted by the Indonesian Transport Society between June and July 2020 found that 209 respondents (45.2 percent) were active public transportation users. Of these active public transportation users, 66 percent are keen on using the service when the pandemic is under control, either in full or with reduced frequency. Furthermore, the survey does not suggest that income alone predicts mode choice. Access to cheap motorcycles offers a possible explanation (JICA, 2019: 37–40, 56–8).

Since July 2020, transit services have been returning to pre-pandemic normal levels in phases. A mild increase in ridership sends a mixed message. After months of revenue loss, growth in ridership numbers is an encouraging sign of recovery. It would be difficult to fully assess the risk of outbreaks among riders until robust testing and tracing strategies are in place. However, of many infection clusters reported in Jakarta since the June 2020 relaxation, not one has been convincingly linked to public transportation use. Instead, risks of infections are linked to the workplace and religious gatherings.[3]

The COVID-19 pandemic and the recession that it induced make Jakarta's pre-existing condition worse. For starters, the government expects that 5.5 million of the country's workforce, dominated by those working in the informal sector, will lose their jobs this year following the slowdown in economic activity. These informal sector workers are more likely to be of lower income and housed mainly in the kampungs.

Conclusion

The COVID-19 pandemic serves as a rear-view mirror. The way it has been handled speaks volumes of the quality of our institutions and the competence of our governments. In the second week of September 2020, Jakarta re-imposed large-scale social restrictions after a marked regression in what was meant to be a period of transition to normality where economic activity can resume in full while observing health and safety protocols. Surging infection and hospitalization rates imply that Jakarta shut down too late and reopened too soon.

A decade worth of public transportation improvements and access to cheap motorcycles have reduced socio-economic inequality in transportation access. Our recent online survey of 462 respondents does not suggest that income alone predicts mode choice. Furthermore, 66 percent of active public transportation users are keen on using the service either in full or with reduced frequency, as soon as the pandemic is under control. On the other hand, a 2018 JICA survey found that eight in nine households (89 percent) own at least one motorcycle and that ownership is equally distributed across income levels (JICA, 2019: 39–40). While the omnipresence of motorcycles offers mixed interpretations, high-quality public transportation seems to have improved transportation equity and therefore mobility justice in Jakarta.

Access to fixed income jobs appeared to be the most consequential pre-existing socio-economic inequality issue during this pandemic. Those without one, that is, those earning daily wages

Pandemic- and Future-Proofing Cities: Pedestrian-oriented Development as an Alternative Model to Transit-based Intensification Centers

Neluka Leanage and Pierre Filion

Introduction

Many official smart growth-inspired Canadian plans limit sprawl by mixing land uses, transportation modes, jobs, and residents to create compact, transit-oriented, multi-functional intensification centers enriched with amenities and highly designed public spaces (Ontario Government Ministry of Municipal Affairs and Housing, 2019 [2006]; City of Toronto, 2018). However, these intensification strategies, built on new or expanded public transit systems at metropolitan, regional, and local planning scales, face challenges amid the 2020 pandemic (Filion et al, 2016).

Recovery from the combined COVID-19-induced loss of commercial activity in intensification centers and confidence in public transit could take years, and combined with an increased reliance on private vehicles, could undo decades of planning efforts at shifting unsustainable land use-transportation dynamics. Concurrently, there is growing attention on sustainable cities with ample public spaces where safe walking and cycling can flourish. Advocates call for reclaiming the streets for people, pedestrians, and cyclists as a resilient strategy for cities and healthy living (Ewing, 2020a). Cities like Milan, Paris, New York, and Seattle are making permanent, temporary space accommodations to pandemic-related pedestrian flows and distancing (Laker, 2020).

This chapter is based on the Canadian (and to a large extent North American) urban reality, which is dominated by low-density, functionally-specialized, and automobile-oriented land uses. Over the last decades, planning efforts to modify this urban form took the form of high-density intensification centers focused on existing or new public transit rail or BRT (bus rapid transit) systems. Such a strategy faces mounting uncertainty amid pandemic-induced, and possibly long-lasting, transit ridership, brick and mortar retailing, and office work decline. We propose as an alternative, or complementary, intensification approach, a pedestrian-oriented development (POD) model inspired by the '15-minute city' being considered across the world. The chapter refers to transit-oriented developments and other attempts at concentrating density and multifunctionality as intensification centers. Different forms of intensification centers share as an objective the creation of spaces that contrast with the North American low-density car-dependent norm. One version of intensification centers discussed here is primarily transit-oriented while the other is more focused on a pedestrian-hospitable environment.

The impacts of COVID-19 on transit-based intensification centers

COVID-19 impacts multiple facets of intensification centers organized around transit and amplifies issues present prior to the pandemic. Fear of contagion has caused apprehension about urban density and transit as well as uncertainty about future planning for intensification. These circumstances call for new ways of making a case for, and delivering, intensification. With increasing evidence of airborne viral transmission, there appears to be sound scientific reasons to avoid large concentrations of people in closed indoor spaces such as bars, lecture halls, theaters, offices, public transit, and airplanes, even when distancing and mask-wearing are practiced (Brosseau, 2020). The reduced use of public transit reflects contagion concerns. Ridership patterns from Toronto, Canada's largest metropolis, indicate that subways servicing the financial center operate below capacity, as a high proportion of office work is done from home (Toronto Transit Commission (TTC), 2020); meanwhile in predominantly racialized, COVID-vulnerable neighborhoods of Toronto, anxiety is high for captive riders employed in the health and service sectors due to crowded buses (CBC News, 2020a). While post-lockdown car use has recovered, transit still struggles with the loss of key passenger markets and pressures to alleviate crowding with sufficient service even as fare revenues have plummeted (TTC, 2020).

Changes in office work patterns may last, impacting public transit use, especially in large metropolitan regions where downtown and its office towers constitute the main transit market. Such shifts can trigger a chain effect percolating through the activity ecology of downtowns and other high-density centers. For example, in Downtown Toronto the underground pedestrian corridor system and its shops and restaurants, which were swamped with office workers during the day, have been nearly empty since the onset of the pandemic.

The capacity of intensification centers to compete with other, lower-density and mostly monofunctional urban districts rested in interconnections between their land uses generating sustainable transportation-based synergy effects. Intensification centers, where much employment was office-based and transit was an important source of accessibility, have been disproportionately

Increased local restaurant patronage and home-based socializing have pulled activities into outdoor public open space and around the home. A high level of neighborhood-based animation over the summer 2020 may be threatened by a COVID-19 resurgence across Canada and the possible reintroduction of restrictions on indoor activities, which would coincide with colder weather, and on social encounters in general.

Polycentric pedestrian-oriented neighborhoods around transit-based intensification centers: an alternative model

Although we cannot anticipate the full consequences of the pandemic on urban trends, we observe a shift in the scales of urban activities from COVID-19 impacts on public transit, intensification centers and the neighborhood public realm (public open spaces but also public and private establishments that are accessible to the public) pointing to a growing importance of the hyperlocal level. As downtown areas lose much of their animation with more people working and studying from home, combined with the avoidance of public transit and indoor commercial facilities, some of the pre-COVID-19 consumption that once occurred in centers is happening in neighborhoods. This is especially the case of downtown restaurants, bars, and gyms, which have suffered a substantial business decline, while similar activities operating at the neighborhood level tend to be performing much better. To adapt to the decline in transit patronage, office work and brick and mortar retailing in intensification centers, and to prevent a rebound of automobile trips, we propose to focus on the public realm at the neighborhood scale, in order to encourage active modes of transportation, catalyze intensification, and replace car trips.

Carlos Moreno (2019) proposed a pedestrian-oriented form of activity distribution for Paris, labeled the 15-minute city. Such a model is inspired by numerous planning concepts including socialist cities' micro-districts, the Garden City, the Jacobian neighborhood and New Urbanist settlements. It entails configuring and coordinating everyday activities so they are accessible within a 15-minute perimeter on foot from any residential location, including: work, shopping, restaurants, entertainment, culture, and education. Larger commercial and government services catering to greater populations, such as health care, libraries, and sport facilities would be accessible within a 30-minute walking territory. Moreno described the 15-minute city as providing hyper-proximity to high-quality living, linking the two essential components of urban life: space and time. By reducing the need for long journeys and hence reliance on motorized transportation, the 15-minute city can compensate for trips diverted from public transit during the pandemic and prevent a surge in automobile use (Sisson, 2020). The 15-minute city emphasizes: high accessibility to amenities as well as high-quality place-based strategies and public realm designs meant for slower movement and outdoor activities such as walking, standing, and sitting. This pedestrian-oriented model differs from the longstanding automobile-oriented neighborhood planning models with residences bound within arterial roads suited to faster and longer travel to reach amenities further afield.

A 15-minute neighborhood embraces walking and engaging in the outdoor public realm, even in colder and wetter weather, by relying on density, infrastructure, and programming. Policies, design, and new technologies can extend the time people can comfortably spend outdoors. A range of innovations to weatherproof PODs could come in the form of municipal responsibility for sidewalk and cycle lane snow-clearing using right-sized equipment, building raincoats like those proposed by Sidewalk Labs' Toronto Quayside project, expandable, modular heated sidewalks and patios, neighborhood-based sheltered outdoor markets, and winter activity promotions and events. In doing so, people can conduct daily activities within walking proximity (Handy and Clifton, 2001) and spend more time outside shopping, dining, exercising, entertaining, and socializing while avoiding the risks of indoor COVID-19 transmission. Creating the conditions for such multifunctional, pedestrian-oriented neighborhoods requires greater emphasis on attracting moderate-to-high-density residential development, supporting safe non-motorized transportation, and animating the public realm, particularly in northern autumn, winter, and spring seasons (Filion et al, 2018).

Such a POD model should be seen as an accompaniment to, and recovery plan for, TOD intensification centers, stretching the common, walkable 800m transit catchment and developable area to 1200m for everyday destinations (a 15-minute walk) and up to 2,400m (30-minute walk) for larger uses, requiring bigger catchment areas. These larger areas could be shared with adjacent PODs, creating a polycentric neighborhood model surrounding and supporting under-serviced and transit-based centers.

As a short term measure, when ridership declines during the pandemic, PODs can provide a transit substitute to sustain attractiveness of intensification centers. In this context, POD can be achieved through a quick adaptation of land use to walking and the animation of intensification centers through public space and pop-up activity. Depending on the time it takes for transit ridership to recover, POD can evolve as an alternative way to support intensification or as a complement to the part public transit plays in this regard.

Implications of the polycentric pedestrian-oriented development (POD) model

To adapt intensification strategies to a polycentric POD model would be a compromise and alternative advancement in the face of uncertainty. The compromise largely supports municipal, regional, and provincial intensification objectives while anticipating what seem to be permanent shifts with deep psychological, behavioral, and recessionary impacts, the recovery from which may take years. While pandemic-related behavior best suited to PODs can promote sustainable mobility, in the longer term as transit recovers and urban centers are reimagined, transit can re-capture active travel users if they have not become reliant on cars. In addition, urban residents desiring amenity-rich, walkable neighborhoods with more space, would not need to leave the city (Foran, 2020). POD can provide alternatives to public transit use and driving, thus reducing the risks of transit-induced contagion and the congestion and environmental sequels of driving, while maximizing near-by accessibility through walking and other outdoor opportunities.

References

Brosseau, L. (2020) 'COVID-19 transmission messages should hinge on science'. *Centre for Infectious Disease Research and Policy, University of Minnesota*, March 16. www.cidrap.umn.edu/news-perspective/2020/03/commentary-COVID-19-transmission-messages-should-hinge-science

CBC News (2020a) *Toronto commuters from communities at high risk for COVID-19 left with little choice*, September 18. www.cbc.ca/player/play/1791585347716

CBC News (2020b) Online shopping has doubled during the pandemic, Statistics Canada says. *Business*, July 24. www.cbc.ca/news/business/online-shopping-covid-19-1.5661818#:~:text=iStock%2FGetty%20Images)-,Canadian%20consumers%20flocked%20to%20online%20shopping%20as%20lockdowns%20to%20combat,to%20a%20Statistics%20Canada%20report.&text=Statistics%20Canada%20says%20e%2Dcommerce,per%20cent%20increase%20over%20February

City of Toronto (2018) *2018 Official Plan – Growth Management Strategy.* www.toronto.ca/city-government/council/2018-council-issue-notes/official-plan-growth-management-strategy/

Ewing, L. (2020a) *Growing calls to re-open parks, expand streets to pedestrians amid COVID-19*, April 18. www.ctvnews.ca/health/coronavirus/growing-calls-to-re-open-parks-expand-streets-to-pedestrians-amid-COVID-19-1.4901999

NINETEEN

Mercurial Images of the COVID-19 City

Emma Arnold

Introduction

Sick city. Quarantine city. Hostile city. Anxious city. Fearful city. Unsafe city. Restrictive city. Dystopian city. Lockdown city. Timeless city. Closed city. Empty city. Isolated city. Distanced city. Divorced city. Pod city. Lonely city. Homeless city. Unequal city. Divided city. Sourdough city. No toilet paper city. Quiet city. Birds are back city. Nature takes over city. Opera on the balcony city. Clapping in the streets city. Work from home city. Zoom city. Frontline city. Essential workers city. Home-schooled city. Unemployed city. Business as usual city. Masked city. Gloved city. Disinfectant city. Plexiglas and tape city. Bored city. Impatient city. Crowded city. Protest city. Compliant city. Defiant city. Selfish city. Selfless city. New normal city.

Multiple and mutable images of the city have emerged during the COVID-19 pandemic. There is the *conceptual image of the city* formed in our imaginations: a newly hostile and restrictive space that influences our affective experiences, emotions, mental health, and behavior. There is the *perceptual image of the city* that has aesthetically and materially changed: redesigned and reconfigured, marked with new materials and by novel forms of litter. These conceptual and perceptual images are in turn forged through the new images *in* and *of* the city that we encounter and create. There are the *images in the city*: signs that instruct us how to act, messages hung in windows, and diverse forms of graffiti and street art. There are the *images of the city*: photographs that document these changing forms, atmospheres, and aesthetics of space. This chapter examines the relationship between image and city during the COVID-19 pandemic and reflects on these mercurial images: images in flux that reflect and communicate different aspects and stages of the pandemic. Referring to photographs taken in Oslo, Norway between March and October 2020, this chapter asks: How does the COVID-19 city look? What is the image of the COVID-19 city? How do these images and pandemic aesthetics impact our urban imaginations?

Image and city

The image of the city can be understood in different ways. Image may refer to the visual matter that makes up the city, from symbols and signs to structures and design. Images can also refer to an impression that one has of place: abstract, imagined, affective, aesthetic, intuited. When considering the relationship between image and city, Kevin Lynch's pivotal book *The Image of the City* is a logical point of departure. Lynch's influential book written in 1960 is largely concerned with visual form, focusing on patterns inherent to the city. It is at once a typology and mediation on the city as an object made up of components and is concerned with how architecture and urban planning influences our image of the city. Though the book is more a practical and technical exploration of what comprises the image of the city – one that is ever-changing and perhaps never fully realized – Lynch acknowledges that 'nothing is experienced by itself, but always in relation to its surroundings, the sequences of events leading up to it, the memory of past experiences' (Lynch, 1960: 1).

Mona Domosh investigates different understandings of 'urban imagery' and offers a more cultural and humanistic interpretation: 'the city, like a painting, is a representation, an image formed out of the hopes and ideas of the cultural worlds in which we live' (Domosh, 1992: 475). Domosh, referring to Lowenthal, argues that the image of the city is more than perceptions and 'reflections of reality' but also 'the result of an active imagination' (Domosh, 1992: 476). Urban photography is another way through which we create and understand the image of the city. Jane Tormey writes that photographs 'say as much about what we imagine cities to be or what we consider to be important about cities, as literature or theory do' (Tormey, 2012: 244). There is no one direct route then to explore the image of the COVID-19 city. What follows is an exploration of some ways to think about the connections, moving from the more abstract conceptual city of our imaginations to the more literal images of the city.

Conceptual and perceptual images of the city

In his book *Landscapes of Fear*, human geographer Yi-Fu Tuan (1979: 102) asks: 'How did a city devastated by pestilence look?' Tuan offers some indications of the image of a city marked by infectious disease, describing scenes from various outbreaks throughout human history. From the typhus epidemic in Athens in 430 BC to the plague in 17th-century London, these descriptions are gruesome and harrowing. Describing the London epidemic of 1665, Tuan writes: 'None could go into the streets without encountering people carrying coffins. There were few passers–by, but of those that one could see, many had sores on them. Others limped painfully from the effects of sores not wholly healed. In silent streets, the red cross flamed upon doors, the few dwellings not so marked being left tenantless and open to the winds' (Tuan, 1979: 103). This stark imagery of past

Figure 19.2: Nets arranged to discourage use at Ekebergsletta football fields in Oslo, March 2020

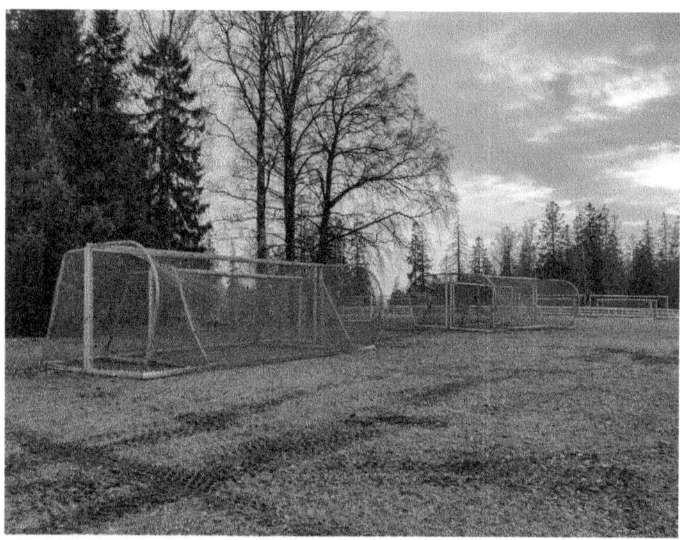

Source: Emma Arnold

Figure 19.3: A view into the Faculty of Social Sciences cafeteria at the University of Oslo where crosses made with masking tape on tables encourage social distancing, September 2020

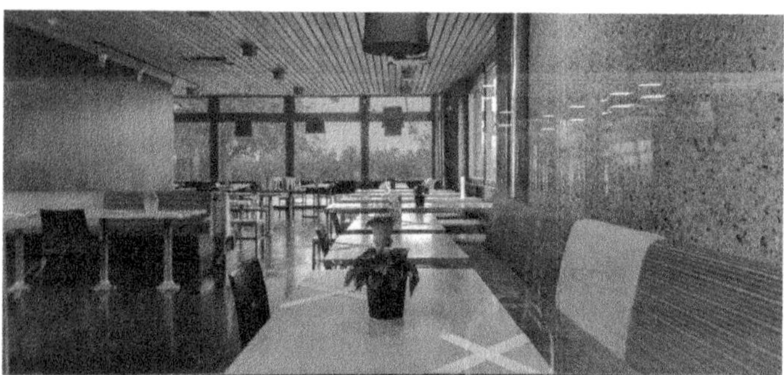

Source: Emma Arnold

Figure 19.4: A disposable mask discarded among leaf litter, October 2020

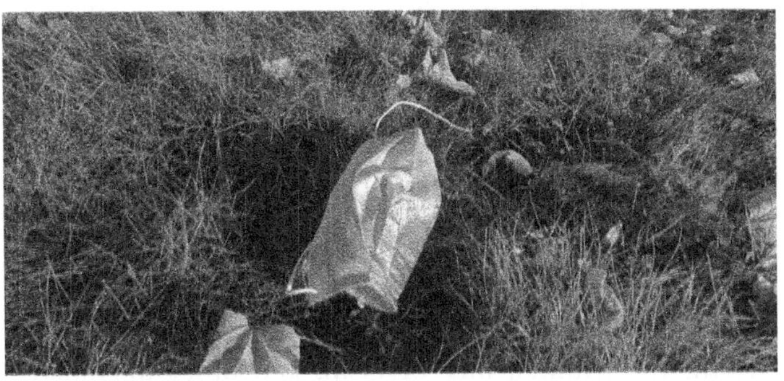

Source: Emma Arnold

The newly masked and socially distanced stranger or the conspicuously unmasked stranger who does not respect social distancing have both become part of the changed urban landscape, giving rise to different affective experiences. Mask-wearing is about public health and slowing rates of transmission but also about optics. Wearing a mask signals that one cares for one's own health as well as the health of others and that one trusts government and science. Masks and gloves have become customary sartorial additions during our daily navigations, and in many places have been made mandatory by authorities. They are also an ubiquitous new form of litter (Figure 19.4). The optics of mask-wearing has become part of policing and protest in public space. In Oslo, the Black Lives Matter demonstration in June and the Extinction Rebellion Oslo Uprising in September are two examples where many activists volunteered to wear masks and other protective gear. While the use of masks is also a matter of protection, it is also to signal responsibility and to ensure that political messages are not undermined by the optics of not wearing masks or worse, a subsequent spike in infection rates.

Images in and of the city

Images inserted into the city and images taken of the city are part of our shifting conceptions and perceptions of urban space. In the newly empty spaces of the city, Young (2020: 1) writes that 'the material infrastructures of lockdown became highly visible'. These material infrastructures include new signs advising not to push buttons at pedestrian crossings and outdoor advertising displays replaced with advice from public health authorities. Official infographic signs from the Norwegian Institute of Public Health, The Norwegian Directorate of Health, the Municipality of Oslo, and other unaffiliated signage appear throughout the city in different formats and spaces (Figures 19.5 and 19.6). The messages are most often reminders on social distancing, hand sanitizing, orders to stay home if ill, and more recently requirements for masks on public transportation. The fear of other people that Tuan (1979) describes during epidemics may be reinforced by these new images in the city. Whether we perceive a given space as safe or not may rely on these changing images. An absence of these images may subsequently lead one to feel unsafe or may

Figure 19.5: Multiple signs on social distancing and hygiene from The Norwegian Directorate of Health and the Norwegian Institute of Public Health hang inside and outside of a small shop, October 2020

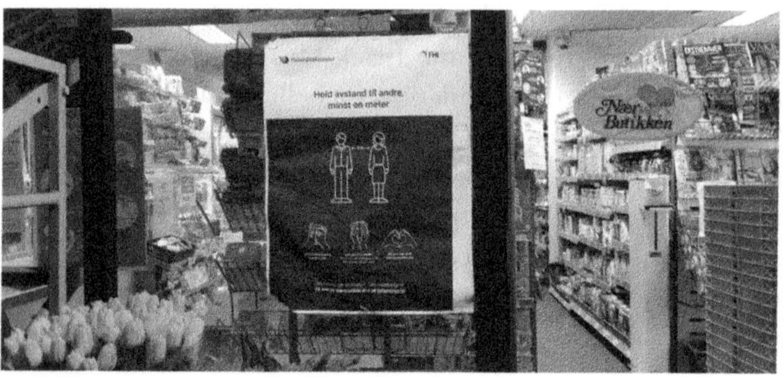

Source: Emma Arnold

Figure 19.6: Municipality of Oslo sign advocating social distancing in queues with small text 'Do it for Oslo' in the lower right corner, September 2020

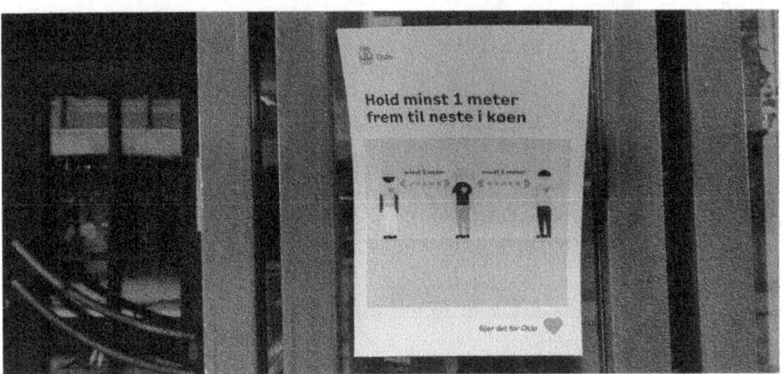

Source: Emma Arnold

serve as an indicator that some kind of 'normal' has returned. Ebbs and flows in these images have been particularly visible on public transportation whose operators have experimented with various ways of minimizing transmission during different stages of the pandemic. While most of these official signs are temporary, others appear more permanent such as the metal traffic sign on one of Oslo's ring roads pointing drivers toward the nearest COVID-19 test center (Figure 19.7).

In contrast to the official signs being inserted into the city, the cultural responses of graffiti and street reflect the peculiarities of the pandemic experience. Stefano Bloch reminds us that graffiti is not 'monolithic' and that graffiti concerning COVID-19 'can best be described as diverse in terms of its members' sentiments, with heavy leanings toward conspiratorial perspectives as well as public health preoccupations' (Bloch, 2020: 1). Julia Tulke describes how graffiti and street artists are playing with predominant visual narratives of the pandemic like the hoarding of toilet paper and the ever-present face mask. Other interventions border on public service announcements and remind the viewer to stay at home or to wash their hands

passively consume these images, we also actively create them as individuals and as a collective. Photographs such as those presented in this chapter are part of a global visual narrative that reveal how cities are changed and how we too are changed by these images. They are informative, communicative, evocative, powerful, and they may also be part of how we are building new imaginings of the future.

From new images to new imaginings

Through the multiple, mutable, and mercurial images of the COVID-19 city, new urban imaginings are being formed: both dystopian and utopian. Through the dystopian image, we may conceive of how other global crises may similarly alter urban landscapes and experience. The climate crisis presents many challenges to cities, writes Paul Dobraszczyk (2017), including how we imagine adapting to a city transformed. He explores the connections between imagination, climate change, and future cities and suggests that representations of the future city transformed by climate change play a part in our adaptability and resilience. The image of the COVID-19 city is of a city transformed that also hints at the utopian and the potential for change. The rapid urban transformation spurred by COVID-19 has been realized through policy, individual and collective action, and the introduction of new materials into the city. Tape, paint, and other materials have become important, versatile, and effective means of reconfiguring urban space and influencing behavior. Justin Davidson writes that tape is 'a liberating force, breathing new flexibility into urban infrastructure that is built to resist change' (Davidson, 2020). This reconfiguration of space is an important part of how the image of cities are changing, whether it is to exclude cars and prioritize space for pedestrians and cyclists or to encourage new behaviors like social distancing and community care. If bits of paper and rolls of tape and concern for the public can radically change the image of the city, what more can we change?

Instead of asking only what the image of the COVID-19 city is, we might also ask: what does the city we want to live in look like? What future city do we imagine? How might we achieve these new urban imaginings?

References

Bloch, S. (2020) 'COVID-19 graffiti'. *Crime, Media, Culture,* 17(1): 27–35.

Davidson, J. (2020) 'How do we rethink public space after the pandemic? Start with rolls of tape'. *New York Magazine.* April 17. https://nymag.com/intelligencer/2020/04/how-to-rethink-public-space-after-COVID-19-start-with-tape.html

Dobraszczyk, P. (2017) 'Sunken cities: climate change, urban futures and the imagination of submergence'. *International Journal of Urban and Regional Research,* 41(6): 868–87.

Domosh, M. (1992) 'Urban imagery'. *Urban Geography,* 13(5): 475–80.

Lynch, K. (1960) *The Image of the City.* Cambridge: The MIT Press.

Tormey, J. (2012) *Cities and Photography.* New York: Routledge.

Tuan, Y. (1979) *Landscapes of Fear.* Minneapolis: University of Minnesota Press.

Tulke, J. (2020) 'Face masks, toilet rolls, and PSAs: the graffiti and street art of the coronavirus pandemic'. *Aesthetics of Crisis* (blog), March 17. http://aestheticsofcrisis.org/2020/graffiti-and-street-art-of-the-coronavirus-pandemic/

Young, A. (2020) 'Locked-down city'. *Crime, Media, Culture,* 17(1): 21–5.

TWENTY

Conclusion

Rianne van Melik, Brian Doucet, and Pierre Filion

Over the past decades, the academic debate on public space has been somewhat Janus-faced, with researchers generally expressing one of two considerations (van Melik, 2017). One set of authors has depicted public space as a socially open and accessible space where meeting and interaction occur, tolerance for diversity is enhanced, democratic values prevail, and art, theater, and performance take place (for example, Lofland, 1989; Watson, 2006; Valentine, 2008). Concurrent with this romanticized ideal, other authors express a sense of loss or nostalgia about public space being eroded and hence being under threat (for example, Mitchell, 1995; 2003; Kohn, 2004). In his critique of American urbanism, Michael Sorkin (1992) even went so far as to herald the 'end of public space'. Authors in this second camp have painted a rather pessimistic picture of modern urban life; one that is characterized by neoliberal urban planning, consumerism, restrictive security measures, and social exclusion.

In a similar vein, chapters in this book by a mix of scholars (in law, criminology, geography, sociology, planning, architecture, and so on) have depicted both bleak and promising developments concerning public space and mobility in times of

(Chapter Fourteen), Thai, Dinh, and Nguyen (Chapter Fifteen), and Dillon and Rukmana (Chapter Seventeen) illustrate, the pandemic has equally resulted in growing inequalities in the access to and use of public space and public transit in Asia and the Middle East (that is, India, Vietnam, and Indonesia); something that asks for further scrutiny. Future research will also need to pay attention to public spaces in African and South American contexts, as there is less literature on these places, specifically when it comes to public space.

This volume discussed public space development occurring in the spring and summer of 2020. At the time of writing, the pandemic was still very much affecting citizens around the world, even worsening in most countries as the second wave of contamination hit in the fall. Our approach in this volume and throughout this series has been to avoid speculating about the future of cities, but rather to show how the pandemic has affected existing patterns of urban design, the use of use of public spaces, and inequality. As we have stressed throughout this series, intersectional approaches that do not treat what happens in public space in isolation are necessary in order to fully interpret the impact of the pandemic.

Because we have focused on understanding how new and pre-existing urban inequalities are manifesting themselves in public space, rather than asking too many questions about how future cities will look like, we do not yet know to what extent the observed developments, patterns, and processes will be transformational. Instead, this volume gives some preliminary answers to 'emerging questions' raised by Honey-Rosés et al (2020), regarding, for example, the mainstreaming of health criteria in the design of public space (for example, Chapters Eight and Nine) or the consideration of the needs of vulnerable groups such as the elderly, children, and the homeless (for example, Chapters Five, Six, Ten, Eleven, Twelve, and Thirteen). If anything, the pandemic has revamped the debate about the value and reclaiming of public space that will most certainly extend after the crisis.

References

Blomley, N. (2011) *Rights of Passage. Sidewalks and the Regulation of Public Flow.* Abingdon: Routledge.

Honey-Rosés, J., Anguelovski, I., Chireh, V.K. et al (2020) 'The impact of COVID-19 on public space: an early review of emerging questions – design, perceptions and inequities'. *Cities & Health*, DOI: 10.1080/23748834.2020.1780074

Kohn, M. (2004) *Brave New Neighborhoods: The Privatization of Public Space.* New York: Routledge.

Lingam, L. and Suresh Sapkal, R. (2020) 'COVID-19, physical distancing and social inequalities: are we all really in this together?' *The International Journal of Community and Social Development*, 2(2): 173–90.

Lofland, L.H. (1989) 'Social life in the public realm: a review'. *Journal of Contemporary Ethnography*, 17(4): 453–82.

Low, S. and Smart, A. (2020) 'Thoughts about public space during Covid-19 pandemic'. *City & Society*, 32(1): np.

Mitchell, D. (1995) 'The end of public space? People's park, definitions of the public, and democracy'. *Annals of the Association of American Geographers*, 85(1): 108–33.

Mitchell, D. (2003) *The Right to the City: Social Justice and the Fight for Public Space.* New York: The Guilford Press.

Sorkin, M. (1992) *Variations on a Theme Park: The New American City and the End of Public Space.* New York: Hill and Wang.

Valentine, G. (2008) 'Living with difference: reflections on geographies of encounter'. *Progress in Human Geography*, 32(3): 323–37.

van Melik, R. (2017) 'De januskop van de openbare ruimte'. *Boekman*, (29)111: 14–17.

Watson, S. (2006) *City Publics: The (Dis)Enchantments of Urban Encounters.* London: Routledge.

Index

References to endnotes show both the page number and the note number (for example, 231n3).

15-minute city 37, 95, 192–3

A

absences and the construction of place 59–60
activities of daily living (ADLs) 98, 109–10, 112
aesthetics of the city 199–211
affluent people/areas
  access to green space 89, 135–6
  cycling provision 172, 173
  efforts to reconfigure public space center 28, 30, 78
  gated communities 180
  public transport provision 91
  urban flight 36, 38–9
ageing-in-place 110, 115, 214
Akers, A. 16
Ali, S.H. 17
'all in this together' myth 214
  see also inequality
allotments 113
Altman, I. 57
Amsterdam 3
anti-social behaviors 59
Aptekar, S. 125
Aronson, L. 101
asylum seekers 47–54
Atkinson, R. 48
attachment to place 55, 57–9, 61, 62

austerity 56, 94, 120, 121, 214
Australia 25, 29, 202
auto-burbs 172

B

Barniskis, S.C. 124
beaches
  closure of 29
  older people 102
  privatization of public space 39, 215
  'selfishness' of using 66–7, 72
Beeckmans, L. 43
Belgium 35–45, 47–54
belonging, sense of 110, 147
benches
  memorial 59–60
  smart technology 105
  use of 49, 61, 98, 103
Bhan, G. 16
Biglieri, S. 17, 133
bike lanes/cycling infrastructure 4, 18, 19, 27–9, 90, 169–72, 179–80, 191, 193
  see also cycling
biodiversity 92, 93
Black, Indigenous, and People of Color (BIPOC) 28
  see also race
Black Lives Matter 3, 20, 22, 71, 205

Moriah, A. 70
Morrow, O. 21
motorcycles 179, 180–1, 182, 183
movement, expectation of 4,
  47–54, 62, 159–60
multiculturalism 17, 143
multimodal/multifunctional uses of
  space 79, 104, 144, 145–6,
  147–8, 187, 188, 194
Murray, N.A. 16
mutual aid 21, 156
mutual vulnerabilities, recognition
  of 21

N

nature, contact with 58, 89, 102,
  113–14, 173
negative freedom 70
neighborhood health care
  centers 41–2
neighborhoods, importance
  of 109–10, 112, 115, 191–4
neoliberalism 17, 65–73, 76–7,
  122, 125, 127, 133, 173, 213–14
Netherlands 3, 110–11, 119–29
Netto, V.M. 152
'new normal' 15, 17, 18, 19–22,
  26, 134–6, 207
New York City, US 27, 77, 98,
  103, 188
Nieuwsblad 39
non-essential travel restrictions 39
non-human species 173
Norway 202–3, 204, 205, 206–9

O

observational walking 146
older people *see* elderly people
Oosterlynck, S. 41
Oslo, Norway 202–3, 204,
  205, 206–9
outdoor childhoods 132
outdoor dining 2, 16, 18, 28, 29,
  39, 215
overcrowding 2–3, 37
over-policing 19
Owen, B. 69

P

Paris, France 2, 77, 95, 170,
  188, 192–3
Parker, B. 21
parking 41, 79, 103, 145,
  146, 167–8
parks
  anti-social behaviors 59
  children in 131–41
  closures 28, 56–7
  for exercise 56–7, 87–9, 101–2,
    132–3, 191
  and health 76, 77–8, 81, 89
  historic decline in 56–7
  London, UK 87–96
  management of 81
  multiple functions of 76
  older people 98, 101–2,
    103, 104
  playgrounds 29, 36, 136, 137–8
  pocket parks 88, 89
  private personal trainers using 29
  privatization of public space 215
  public funding of 79, 94, 95
  'selfishness' of using 66–7, 72
  'seniors only' 103, 104
  social distancing 57, 76
  for social interactions 88–9,
    131–2, 137–8, 191–2
  sports in 2
  transport links to 78, 80
  UK 55–64, 87–96
  US 75–83
  see also green public space
participant observation
  methods 144, 146
participatory action research 43
participatory drawings 134
participatory engagement
  methods 27, 81
pavements *see* sidewalks
pedestrianization 26, 28, 79, 103
pedestrian-oriented
  development 187–97
pedestrians 2, 4, 27, 181, 187–97
perceptual images of the
  city 200, 201–5